Bibliotherapy with Young People

Bibliotherapy with Young People

Librarians and Mental Health Professionals Working Together

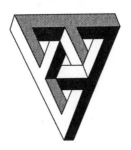

Beth Doll

Associate Professor

Director, School Psychology Program

University of Colorado at Denver

and

Carol Doll

Associate Professor

Graduate School of Library and Information Science

University of Washington

1997
Libraries Unlimited, Inc.
Englewood, Colorado

Libraries Unlimited, Inc.
P.O. Box 6633
Englewood, CO 80155-6633
1-800-237-6124

Production Editor: Stephen Haenel
Copy Editor: Brooke Graves
Proofreader: Lori Kranz
Indexer: Christine Smith
Typesetter: Michael Florman

Library of Congress Cataloging-in-Publication Data

Doll, Beth, 1952-   .
    Bibliotherapy with young people : librarians and mental health
professionals working together / Elizabeth Jane Doll and Carol A. Doll
    vii, 124 p. 17x25 cm.
    Includes bibliographical references and index.
    ISBN 1-56308-407-4
    1. Bibliotherapy for children. 2. Bibliotherapy for teenagers.
I. Doll, Carol Ann, 1949-   . II. Title.
RJ505.B5D65 1997
615.8'516'083--dc21
                                                    96-51730
                                                       CIP

Contents

PREFACE

This book grew out of a series of dinner conversations about the practice of bibliotherapy with children and youth, held over the family table or during holiday reunions. With one of us trained in library and information science and the other a psychologist, these were far-ranging and contentious debates about all facets of the practice: Should bibliotherapy be practiced at all? Who is qualified to be a bibliotherapist? Which children should be targeted? Is the practice effective? (But don't jump to conclusions—the psychologist was far more comfortable with many practices of nonpsychologists than was the media specialist!) We not only disagreed, but we also confused one another with arguments that did not seem consistent with the bibliotherapy practices that we each had experienced. Finally, we realized that we were using very different definitions of the term *bibliotherapy*. Not only that, but very different things occurred during the bibliotherapy programs we were familiar with, with the practices applied to different kinds of children and for different purposes. As our conversations progressed, we realized that we were mimicking the debates in our different professional communities. In the literature, as in our own debates, different authors use different definitions, speak of different children, and presume different activities when they write about bibliotherapy practices. Once we clarified our own definitions and reframed them into a new and broader definition of bibliotherapy, the questions that guided our conversations changed as well. These new questions, which are described in chapter 1, provide the focus around which this book was written.

We had a second realization as well: Although each of us was very comfortable with some facets of bibliotherapy programs, there were aspects that each of us was quite unfamiliar with. The psychologist understands very little about media selection: locating, evaluating, and choosing among different books, films, or media. Alternatively, the media specialist is uncomfortable with her understanding of social and emotional adjustment and the signals that children and adolescents send when a program or discussion is being disruptive rather than helpful. Together, though, we have been able to design and implement programs of bibliotherapy that are far richer than either of us could have developed in isolation. (An example is included as appendix B.) Thus we have come to believe that collaborations between professionals, and in particular collaborations among mental health professionals, media specialists, and children's and young adults' librarians, are the most fruitful strategies for high-quality bibliotherapy programs. Consequently, collaborative practices became the unifying focal point for this book.

1 Introduction

REFRAMING THE QUESTIONS

Simply defined, *bibliotherapy* is sharing a book or books with the intent of helping the reader deal with a personal problem. However simple its definition, the practice of bibliotherapy is difficult to describe, defend, or debate. Indeed, mention the word wherever children's professionals are gathered and a heated discussion is likely to ensue. Some will defend the practice of bibliotherapy as a rich and sensitive strategy for supporting children through the difficult process of growing up. Others will attack bibliotherapists as charlatans who promise to transform children's everyday lives but actually affect them little if at all. Controversies may emerge about the training of bibliotherapists. Some would reserve the title for rigorously trained mental health professionals to the dismay of others, who believe that daily practices of teachers, librarians, and media specialists include legitimate examples of "bibliotherapy." Arguments might be made for protecting children from the unqualified practices of pseudotherapists or, alternatively, for giving troubled children ample access to quality literature presented by caring adults. Whatever the speakers' position, their beliefs about bibliotherapy are invariably passionate and strongly held.

We do not, in this book, take a stand on the prevailing discussion about bibliotherapy and its practice, because we believe these are the wrong issues and that further discussion would be nonproductive. Instead, we reframe the practice of bibliotherapy around certain parameters, including:

- The purposes that bibliotherapists attempt to address using books;
- The degree to which these purposes match the nature and prevalence of the mental health needs of children and young adults;
- Given these purposes and needs, the degree to which programs of bibliotherapy are justified;
- The different skills and competencies provided by different professionals to support such programs.

Within this broad and refocused setting, we redefine the issues by asking questions about the practice of bibliotherapy.

Should Bibliotherapy Be Practiced?

Although frequently asked, this question means different things when asked by different professionals. When librarians and media specialists ask whether bibliotherapy should be practiced, they are frequently asking whether the purpose and responsibilities imposed by the practice of bibliotherapy are outside the scope of the typical library professional. In effect, this becomes our second question—that of who is a qualified bibliotherapist. When mental health professionals ask whether bibliotherapy should be practiced, they are asking whether the practice of bibliotherapy is effective in achieving its intended purpose. This question cannot be answered without first defining bibliotherapy and clarifying its purposes.

Such clarification is the focus of chapter 2, "Bibliotherapy Defined." The chapter begins with a review of the varying and inconsistent definitions of bibliotherapy provided in the professional literature and offers a summative definition of bibliotherapy as a continuum ranging from simple reading guidance to comprehensive programs of psychotherapy. Next, the chapter examines seven different purposes that have been proposed for programs of bibliotherapy. A summary description of activities composing programs of bibliotherapy is provided, together with a description of the competencies children need to benefit from them. Finally, issues of bibliotherapy effectiveness are examined. The annotated bibliography in appendix A directs readers to resources listing useful activities and program structures.

Which Children and Youth Should Be Targeted for Bibliotherapy Programs?

As bibliotherapy moves along the continuum from simple reading guidance to comprehensive therapy programs, its intended audience shifts from typical children with their everyday problems and triumphs toward children with unique needs and emotional vulnerabilities. Thus, depending upon the program and its intent, any child or adolescent could be an appropriate participant in a bibliotherapy program. The more important question, then, is "What kinds of adult support do different groups of children require?" Second, "Does the support provided by a particular program of bibliotherapy match the needs of the children who participate in it?"

Assistance in answering these questions can be found in chapter 3, "Mental Health Needs of Children and Adolescents." The chapter examines three sets of needs: those faced by most typical children as they move through the challenging task of growing up; those faced by children living with economic or social hardships that make them vulnerable to social and emotional problems; and those faced by children and adolescents with significant mental disorders. An underlying message of chapter 3 is that the mental health needs of children and adolescents far outnumber the adults available to provide support. Thus, any adult working with youth is likely to be faced with any or all of these mental health needs, whether or not the adult has specialized mental health training. Consequently, chapter 6, "Cautions for Bibliotherapy Leaders," provides a brief explanation of the signs of distress that might become evident when a vulnerable youth is inadvertently overstressed by an activity, discussion, or book.

Who Should Practice Bibliotherapy?

This question, too, depends heavily upon what is meant by the term *bibliotherapy*. Is bibliotherapy simply an opportunity for adults to provide guidance to youth? In that case, there are many adult professionals who have the training and expertise to interact with children and young adults in all types of settings. Indeed, advising and sharing insight are natural parts of supportive adult-child relationships and are expected skills for adult professionals working with youth. Books and other materials provide a ready vehicle for such mentoring.

Is *bibliotherapy*, instead, another term for matching books to young readers' needs? This function has long been a part of library work with children. Chapter 4, "Skills of the Youth Librarian/Media Specialist," describes the specialized skills that make this profession uniquely suited to match children and books. Librarians and school library media specialists work diligently to find books, videos, tapes, computer programs, CD-ROMs, and other formats that contain the information or entertainment wanted or needed by those who use the collection. They organize these materials and then devote time and energy to matching particular items to individual users. For librarians and media specialists, sharing their own enthusiasm for the ideas, stories, characters, and imagination found in good materials is one of the most important and enjoyable parts of the job.

Furthermore, they need not rely strictly on personal knowledge to select books and media. There are a multitude of reference books designed to help identify the "perfect" match by author, title, subject, type of material, reading level, sequel, or any other quality imaginable. Although familiar to most youth librarians, these references are relatively unknown among mental health professionals. Chapter 7, "Bibliographic Tools," describes selected references and explains how they were chosen for readers unfamiliar with this task.

Is bibliotherapy a form of psychotherapy, with the purpose of treating mental disorders of children and adolescents? If so, it would be irresponsible to conduct such a program without the involvement of a mental health professional. Even this can be confusing, though, as there are many different mental health professions and methods, each with its unique history, traditions, and theoretical models. Chapter 5, "Skills of the Mental Health Professional," describes these professions and their differing titles. Moreover, chapter 5 explains the standards that have emerged for effective programs of therapy for children and youth, and how these programs might be augmented by bibliotherapy components.

WORKING TOGETHER

Because of the unique talents of different professionals, and the complex array of options that bibliotherapy programs provide, this book proposes a partnership among librarians, media specialists, and mental health professionals as the optimal staffing strategy for bibliotherapy programs. For example, youth librarians can work with mental health professionals, using their knowledge of children's and young adult literature to identify appropriate materials. At the same time, the mental health professional can negotiate the oftentimes delicate interaction with children or young adults who are experiencing severe distress. Chapter 8, "Building a Bibliotherapy Program," provides a step-by-step explanation of how to plan and implement such a bibliotherapy program, drawing upon the information and examples of the previous chapters. A special focus of chapter 8 is the negotiation of effective team relationships that permit diverse professionals to share expertise and responsibility. Finally, appendix B describes a sample program that resulted from just such a planning process.

We believe that redefining and reframing these questions about bibliotherapy allows for the development of new approaches to an established practice—approaches that will permit professionals to be more effective when working with children and young adults.

2 Bibliotherapy Defined

Reading through a single article about bibliotherapy is inspiring. Each of us has been struck by the persuasive power of books, at one time or another, and many of us use books to help us make important personal decisions. It only makes sense that we would want to share this same power with the children and adolescents with whom we work. However, reading through several different articles about bibliotherapy leads to confusion. It is immediately evident that different authors use the same term to describe different activities with different kinds of children. In this chapter, we show how much of the controversy surrounding bibliotherapy is due, in part, to these different understandings. We begin with an overview of bibliotherapy as it is described in both the library media and the mental health literature. Various definitions are examined, followed by a description of the purposes for which bibliotherapy is used, and finally by a description of what occurs during different forms of bibliotherapy. Next, because we are examining bibliotherapy with young readers, we discuss the capacities that children and young adults must have to benefit both socially and emotionally from bibliotherapy. Only after clarifying these definitions and descriptions do we examine the question of who should provide bibliotherapy and when. Finally, our attention turns to evidence supporting the effectiveness of bibliotherapy in enhancing the comfort and well-being of children and adolescents.

DEFINITIONS OF BIBLIOTHERAPY

Within the field of library and information science, many authors carefully present an explanation of bibliotherapy in their books or articles. Definitions range from very simple to quite complex and from very broad to narrowly specific. The simplest definitions describe bibliotherapy as the healing power of books. For example, Bernstein (1989, 159) states, "The term 'bibliotherapy,' most simply defined, means helping with books. Everyone can be helped through reading, including those people not currently faced with a problem, not in therapy, and not directed to the reading material by someone else." This same sentiment is echoed in Smith's (1989, 241) definition: "Simply put, [bibliotherapy] can be defined as healing through books." Similarly, Ashley (1987, 220) concludes, "Bibliotherapy, then, may be seen as remediation through reading." The *Dictionary of Education* (Good 1966, 212) provides a lengthier definition: "[U]se of books to influence total development, a process of interaction between the reader and literature which is used for personality assessment, adjustment, growth, clinical and mental hygiene purposes; a concept that ideas inherent in selected reading material can have a therapeutic effect upon the mental or physical ills of the reader." Finally, Hart's (1987–1988, 56) definition states, "In bibliotherapy, the counselor or librarian provides guidance in the solution of personal problems through directed reading."

Other authors use the term *bibliotherapy* only when reading is accompanied by activities specifically planned to help readers draw healing insight from books. For example, Hébert (1991) attributes the success of bibliotherapy to the discussion, role-playing, and creative problem-solving activities that follow the reading of books. Similarly, Pardeck (1994, 1990b) describes five steps that constitute bibliotherapy, including activities to establish rapport and identify the children's special needs before selecting books to be read, and activities that guide children toward insight and extend their understanding of a book's characters after they have read the book. In an even more restrictive definition, Rosen (1987) argues that effective therapy using books must also include plans for implementing children's newfound insight, strategies to monitor their compliance with these plans, and provisions for correcting plans that prove to be ineffective.

Similar inconsistencies exist in descriptions of the targets of bibliotherapy. Whereas Hart (1987–1988, 212) and Bernstein (1989, 159) exclaim, "Everyone can be helped through reading," other authors select only troubled youth to help. Some of the confusion is undoubtedly due to the incorporation of the word *therapy* in *bibliotherapy,* which automatically invokes assumptions that its purpose is to cure illness or treat dysfunction. Indeed, definitions of bibliotherapy include many references to remediation, therapeutic effect, and personal problems, leading one to expect that the children and youth who participate in it are largely a dysfunctional and harried lot. Pardeck (1989a) clarifies this inconsistency by describing three different targets of bibliotherapy: the emotionally troubled, those with minor adjustment problems, and children with typical developmental needs. Extended descriptions of each of these groups can be found in chapter 3.

One more definition of bibliotherapy is found only within the mental health journals. There *bibliotherapy* sometimes refers to the use of self-help books in lieu of face-to-face therapy (Rosen 1987). The targets of self-help bibliotherapy are typically "clients" with identified socioemotional dysfunction. Again, some directions for self-help therapies involve simply giving a book to the parent or youth; other methods incorporate discussions before reading to identify the nature and extent of the problem, ongoing monitoring during reading to assist in application of the book's message and check for compliance, and follow-up services to ensure that the book's recommendations have been implemented successfully.

Some authors have addressed this definitional confusion by specifying types of bibliotherapy. Gladding and Gladding (1991, 12), for instance, call the minimalist definition of bibliotherapy "reactive bibliotherapy" and note that it "has involved the assignment of library materials to children and their hopefully positive reaction to their assignment." They call a second form of bibliotherapy "interactive bibliotherapy" and explain that in this form, "the processes of growth, change, and healing that occur in clients are centered not so much in the reading of material by individuals as in the guided dialogue about the material" (Gladding and Gladding 1991, 78). Hynes (1990, 264) points out that interactive bibliotherapy requires a facilitator to guide the reader's interaction with literature and "uses literature and/or creative writing as a catalyst for growth and healing."

One of the most useful typologies is Lack's (1985) distinction between "developmental bibliotherapy" and "clinical bibliotherapy," based on both the kinds of activities used and the type of child engaged. She explains, "*Developmental bibliotherapy* is the personalization of literature for the purpose of meeting normal ongoing life tasks. *Clinical bibliotherapy* is a mode of intervention in aiding persons severely troubled with emotional or behavioral problems" (Lack 1985, 29). In developmental bibliotherapy, the reading materials and discussions emphasize general personality development; in clinical bibliotherapy, they focus on specific problems. Likewise, Pardeck and Pardeck (1986, 3) describe programs of bibliotherapy that focus on "helping children cope with developmental needs, typical problems that do not need advanced therapeutic intervention."

These diverse and wide-ranging meanings for the term *bibliotherapy* have added confusion to the professional debates about when bibliotherapy is appropriate and who should be doing it. Within this book, we try to unite these varying explanations by considering bibliotherapy as a continuum: At its simplest, it can be the private and personal insight that a child gains from a book or video, whereas the other end of the continuum represents the urgent and complex type of therapy that occurs between the seriously disturbed client and the highly trained mental health professional. To facilitate our dialogue, this book uses Lack's terminology of *developmental bibliotherapy* to refer to the former and her term *clinical bibliotherapy* to refer to the latter extremes of this continuum. In between fall the varying gradations of guided reading that are described in both library media and mental health journals and books. Later in this chapter we describe how to distinguish between programs of bibliotherapy that are essentially developmental and those that are clinical and so require the participation and leadership of a mental health professional.

PURPOSES OF BIBLIOTHERAPY

What do bibliotherapists expect to accomplish through their work? The reasons for doing bibliotherapy are as diverse as its definitions. Indeed, at least seven different purposes can be found scattered among different references describing bibliotherapy. Above all else, bibliotherapy's most common purpose is to foster personal insight and self-understanding among the children and youth who read. Spache (1978, 241) credits other anonymous authorities with saying, "[T]he values of bibliotherapy include the opportunity to learn to know one's self better, to understand human behavior and to find interest outside the self." Bump (1990) describes *insight* more precisely as helping youth identify and articulate the feelings they had while they read. Hynes (1990) also believes that the emotions evoked by reading can lead to integrating self-knowledge. Jeon (1992) describes several different types of insight that emerge from books, including acquired knowledge about the psychology of human behavior, understanding of the basic motivations of persons with problems like one's own, and clarification of the difficulties posed by one's own behavior. Still, the most eloquent description of insight was provided by Bruce Colville (1990, 35), a prominent children's author, when he poetically stated,

> the right story at the right moment is an arrow to the heart. It can find and catch what is hiding inside the reader (or the listener), the secret hurt or anger or need that lies waiting, aching to be brought to the surface.

Second, in a goal closely linked to that of enhancing personal insight, some bibliotherapists seek to trigger an emotional catharsis in the children with whom they work. *Catharsis* is the release of emotional or psychological tension that occurs when readers experience the feelings of the characters about which they read. Corman (cited in Ashley 1987) argues that catharsis purifies readers of tensions and so leaves them better able to recognize themselves in the characters of a book. Others argue that the release of emotional tension is, in and of itself, therapeutic (Chatton 1988; Halsted 1988). Jeon (1992) points out that book-induced emotions are easier for children to cope with and for adults to assist with because they are more predictable and controlled than the spontaneous emotions that children experience otherwise.

As a third purpose, several prominent bibliotherapists argue that literature and film can assist children and adolescents with solving their day-to-day problems. Hendrickson (1988, 40) believes that bibliotherapy "is a valid and reasonable means of attempting to help children learn to cope with the emotional disruptions they may encounter." According to Pardeck and Pardeck (1986, 1), "[l]iterature can be used as an effective tool for helping children cope with developmental change." Sullivan (1987, 875) writes about using literature to explore sensitive issues with her students. "[T]he purpose for this program was not to entertain pupils, but to use carefully selected books as a catalyst for discussion in the hope of sensitizing her pupils to current social concerns and helping them seek solutions to their own problems." Jeon (1992, 17) advocates using bibliotherapy with gifted children for similar reasons, saying, "[B]ibliotherapy can be very useful in helping gifted children resolve their personal, academic, and/or career problems." A vivid explanation of how literature assists problem solving is provided by Frasier and McCannon (1981) when they suggest that readers are permitted, through imagination, to try out various solutions without suffering the real-life consequences. Similarly, Hébert (1991) notes that through books children and adolescents can thoughtfully analyze a problem situation while remaining safe from the consequences of their imagined decisions. Fictional works might assist children both by posing solutions to problems that readers had not considered independently or by describing consequences of those solutions that readers had not anticipated (Jeon 1992; Pardeck and Pardeck 1984a).

Fourth, most bibliotherapists also believe that the insight, catharsis, and assistance with problem solving provided by literature will cause young people to change the ways in which they interact with or behave toward other people. For example, Gladding and Gladding (1991, 7) indicate that "[t]he premise underlying this approach was that clients' identification with literary characters similar to themselves was helpful in releasing emotions, gaining new directions in life, and promoting new ways of interacting." Some argue that the impact of books will be short-lived unless bibliotherapists prompt these behavioral shifts toward more productive and beneficial actions (Lack 1985). Thus, the emergence of behavior changes represents the ultimate test of the utility and effectiveness of bibliotherapy.

A fifth purpose of bibliotherapy is the promotion of effective and satisfying relationships with other people. Chatton (1988) explains that children gain a sense of connectedness with the groups with which they read and share books. Lack (1985) also comments on the importance of the stimulation and sharing that take place within book discussion groups. Books can provide a focus around which shared interests and common experiences can be discovered, and so can provide a foundation for future friendships. In a related purpose, books can diminish personal isolation by allowing readers to recognize themselves in the characters of fiction. Halsted (1988) calls this the purpose of "universalization" and points out the importance of recognizing that the difficulties one faces are not solely one's own. The awareness that others have faced similar problems may be the first step toward recognizing that the problems are solvable.

Sixth, bibliotherapy may act as a source of information for youth when they face specific problems that set them apart from their peers. For example, Coleman and Ganong (1990, 327) use literature involving stepfamilies with both adults and young people. They indicate that "[b]ibliotherapy is a helpful method for informing stepchildren and their parents about steprelationships and the unique challenges they may encounter." Pardeck described similar applications of bibliotherapy for several distinct groups, including foster care (1990a), blended families (1989a), and adoption (1989b). Anderson (1992, 83) discusses the use of bibliotherapy with chronically ill children in a pediatric setting. She says, "With the firm belief that chronically ill, hospitalized young patients are children first, we can use books to enable and empower them to become enriching participants in a multicultural society."

Seventh, and often overlooked, are the recreational purposes underlying bibliotherapy: Children and youth also read for the enjoyment that reading brings. Indeed, Chatton (1988) describes recreation as the primary purpose of bibliotherapy. Gubert (1993, 127) also acknowledges recreational purposes when she says, "Practitioners aim to alleviate boredom or a sense of futility in patients by helping them develop new interests to promote personal growth and new ways to behave." Indeed, the attractiveness of literature and film can be a principal contribution of bibliotherapy to the therapeutic process.

Summary

This list of seven purposes is not meant to be exhaustive. Indeed, there may be as many purposes to bibliotherapy as there are professionals who use it. A more important question is whether these purposes can be successfully achieved. The answer to this question depends, in part, on the strategies used by the bibliotherapist to introduce, read, and examine the book with young readers.

WHAT OCCURS DURING BIBLIOTHERAPY

Given the diverse definitions of bibliotherapy, and the different purposes that bibliotherapists have set out, it is not surprising to find differing accounts of the activities that constitute bibliotherapy programs. Certain descriptions of how to "do" bibliotherapy are rather brief and sketchy. For example, Hendrickson (1988, 40) speaks briefly about matching the appropriate book to the individual child and following up to evaluate the suitability of that match. Other descriptions are more extensive. For example, Lack (1985) shares the ground rules used in her groups and gives examples of specific activities she has used successfully. Jeon (1992), in contrast, offers a list of twelve ways to implement bibliotherapy suggested by other authors. Chatton (1988) provides a shorter but more detailed list of guidelines for bibliotherapy. Gladding and Gladding (1991) offer practical steps to follow when initiating bibliotherapy in schools. Sullivan (1987) gives tips on involving parents, selecting materials, conducting read-aloud sessions, and leading discussions. (To assist professionals in designing their own program of bibliotherapy activities, we have assembled these and other references into an annotated bibliography of resources; see appendix A.)

Drawing upon these and other authors, Pardeck (1994) constructed a four-step model of clinical bibliotherapy, whereas Jeon (1992) described a three-step model of developmental bibliotherapy. The two models are very similar. In table 2.1, we have combined them into a single model of bibliotherapy in which developmental bibliotherapy incorporates three activities: material selection, material presentation, and comprehension-building activities. Clinical bibliotherapy includes these three steps plus two more: readiness activities, which precede the selection of reading materials, and follow-up and evaluation activities, which represent a long-term follow-up to verify that the problem has been solved. Descriptions of particular recommendations that different authors have made for bibliotherapy can be referenced to these five steps.

Table 2.1. Activities Comprising Each Step in Developmental and Clinical Bibliotherapy

Step	Developmental Bibliotherapy	Clinical Bibliotherapy
Readiness	This step is not included in developmental bibliotherapy	• Establishing rapport with the client • Agreeing together on what the problem is • Exploring the extent and precise nature of the problem • Conducting additional assessment of the child's condition, as needed
Material Selection	• Selecting high-quality books that match the young person's reading level and interest • Selecting books (and other media) that build upon the young person's current understanding	• Selecting high-quality books that match the young person's reading level and interest • Selecting materials that build upon the young person's current understanding of the previously identified problem • Selecting materials that offer an explanation of the presenting problem that is compatible with the client's present understanding • Selecting materials that offer solutions that are likely to be successful in the client's situation

Step	Developmental Bibiotherapy	Clinical Bibliotherapy
Presentation of Materials	• Suggesting the book in a way that enhances the young person's interest in it • Perhaps punctuating the reading with interrupting activities designed to enhance comprehension	• Suggesting the book in a way that enhances the young person's interest in it • Perhaps punctuating the reading with interrupting activities designed to enhance comprehension • Monitoring and defusing excessive distress or unhealthy emotional responses to the book
Comprehension-Building	• Assisting young readers in examining the principal characters and problems of the book • Giving special attention to the motivations that lead characters to act in certain ways • Pointing out the problems that are examined within the book's plot, the solutions that are posed, and the consequences of different solutions • Helping participants see similarities between the book's characters and themselves or people they know	• Assisting young readers in examining the principal characters and problems of the book • Giving special attention to the motivations that lead characters to act in certain ways • Pointing out the problems that are examined within the book's plot, the solutions that are posed, and the consequences of different solutions • Helping participants see similarities between the book's characters and themselves or people they know
Follow-Up and Evaluation	• This step is not included in developmental bibliotherapy	• Prompting the young person's decision to take action • Assisting young readers in developing a reasonable action plan that is likely to be successful • Monitoring the action plan over time to ensure that it is being followed • Revising and reattempting action plans as often as needed to see effects

Readiness activities represent one of two steps that set clinical bibliotherapy apart from developmental bibliotherapy. When working with children and adolescents who have significant mental health needs, a clinical bibliotherapist first works to establish an effective rapport with the child or adolescent and the child's family. Then, using this rapport, the therapist identifies and systematically analyzes the reasons underlying the family's decision to seek therapy. These reasons might be problems with the child's behavior or coping skills, or may be problems of traumatic life changes that the child is facing. A more extensive description of this problem exploration process appears in chapter 3. In either case, the problems identified within these readiness activities, and the assessment of the child's perspective on and understanding of the problems, become the focus for subsequent bibliotherapy activities. Thus, accurate identification of the presenting problems is of paramount importance if the clinical bibliotherapy activities are to be effective.

Material selection. Selection of the right book or film can heighten the interest of the children and young adults who participate, or can guarantee the program's failure. An extensive discussion of the criteria describing high-quality children's literature is included in chapter 4; also, Pardeck and Pardeck (1986) provide a list of specific criteria to be applied to books for the preschool child. In addition to the literary quality of the material, bibliotherapists select books on the basis of their match with the problems and life experiences of the program's participants. Clinical bibliotherapists, in particular, seek materials that have therapeutic utility for a particular child; toward this end, they choose materials that provide information about the actual problem or problems with which a child is faced, offer a perspective of the problem that is likely to be useful given the child's own life situation, and furnish perspectives that are only slightly more sophisticated than the child's own understanding of the problem.

Presentation of materials. Selected books can be read either aloud or silently. Silent reading can occur within the larger group or independently, at the child's own pace. Books read aloud can be interrupted with discussion questions, punctuated with films or illustrations, acted out, or read through cover-to-cover without interruption. Films, too, can be shown in a single sitting, or interrupted and punctuated with discussions or application activities. When interruptions occur, Pardeck (1994) suggests that they be used to help participants see the similarities between themselves and the book's characters, to debrief emotional responses that they have had to the book, or to analyze the problems being faced by characters and the options the characters have for solving them. In fact, Dreyer (1989) describes the insight, catharsis, and identifications that occur while material is being presented as the principal features of bibliotherapy. Presenting the material within the group makes it possible to examine the readers' emotional experiences as they emerge.

Comprehension-building activities. Whether or not the presentation has been interrupted with discussions, subsequent comprehension activities provide opportunities for readers to reflect upon the book, including the problems that were addressed, the characters that emerged, the characters' similarities to and differences from the reader, the human motivations that were described, and the applications these motivations have for the readers' own lives. When discussions are used to elaborate upon a book or film, Cianciolo (1965) suggests the following format:

1. Retell a story emphasizing incidents, feelings, relationships, values, and behaviors
2. Identify similar events from the reader's life
3. Explore the consequences that occurred
4. Generalize the consequences of certain behaviors
5. Evaluate the helpfulness of different alternatives.

Bump (1990) uses a different approach of character analysis to support his bibliotherapy program on substance abuse. He asks his students to select the characters they most admire, who are most often the book's sober characters. Alternatively, after identifying the substance-abusing characters in a book, Bump will ask students to list characteristics of substance dependency, or he will assign self-help books in addition to a literary work and give students the task of applying self-help principles to the characters. Bump also uses a two-column journaling procedure so that his students can reference their reflections to key passages in a book. On occasion, he uses a synchronous computer network to permit anonymous discussion of a work within a class. Bernstein (1989) considers the discussion portion of bibliotherapy so important that she dedicates more than four pages of her article to giving discussion guidelines, talking about preparing for the discussion, and suggesting self-examination questions for professionals.

Comprehension activities need not be limited to group discussions. Pardeck (1994, 1990b) provides several ideas for graphic or dramatic follow-up activities to reinforce participants' understanding of the books. For example, he describes creative writing activities in which the student assumes the role of the character, art activities in which students draw key scenes or characters in a book, role-playing activities that replay key decisions one character makes, or mock trials in which ethical and legal perspectives of a single incident in a book are debated.

Follow-up and evaluation are culminating activities of clinical bibliotherapy. They are meant to ensure that readers' new insights and understandings are translated into meaningful changes in their lives. Thus, a critical step of follow-up is to assist children or young adults in deciding to address their problems as a result of the bibliotherapy and to help them devise realistic action plans to do so. Still, the best of intentions fade quickly once a bibliotherapy program has ended, making a second critical feature of this stage the ongoing monitoring of the action plan to ensure that the child is following it. Lapsed action plans may be a sign that the child has lost interest, but may also signal a problem with the plan or its effectiveness. Clinical bibliotherapists will work with the child to revise and retry action plans as many times as necessary to make them effective. Finally, a clinical bibliotherapist will check back with the child after several weeks or months to ensure that the benefits of the bibliotherapy have been lasting. These final activities of clinical bibliotherapy are virtually indistinguishable from other programs of child therapy (described in more detail in chapter 3).

Summary

As can be seen from the preceding brief descriptions, there are many things to consider when preparing for bibliotherapy: the audience, the program's purpose, and the program's position on the continuum between developmental and clinical bibliotherapy. Moreover, a fourth important decision must be made about who should be involved. When a program is clearly developmental in its intent and targeted audience, bibliotherapists can be more flexible in deciding whom to involve and how. Depending on the type of session planned and the nature of the problems to be confronted, librarians, teachers, media specialists, mental health personnel, or other professionals may work individually or collaboratively. When a program is clearly clinical, involvement of mental health specialists is mandatory. In either case, collaboration among and within professions can only strengthen a carefully planned session with young people. Chapter 8 gives guidance by describing the options for collaboration that bibliotherapists might use and the range of and standards for collaborative techniques.

WHAT CHILDREN NEED TO
BENEFIT FROM BIBLIOTHERAPY

Before literature can become an instrument of change in young readers' lives, they must have the intellectual sophistication needed to use that instrument effectively. In particular, young readers must have three important skills to benefit from bibliotherapy programs. First, bibliotherapy relies on children's abilities to imagine, however briefly, what it must be like to live in the world of the character. It is by "walking a mile in the character's moccasins" that young readers gain key insights into the experiences, feelings, and behaviors of persons other than themselves. Second, children must have rudimentary social problem-solving skills to use the insight they gain through bibliotherapy. Simple problem-solving skills include being able to describe the problem clearly, to see more than one possible solution, and to systematically evaluate the different solutions when choosing among them. These steps allow young readers to fit the problems, solutions, and consequences found in literature into a plan for personal action. Third, young readers must be purposeful in changing their own behavior to bring it into line with their newfound plan of action. Unless they can set and work toward personal goals, the insight that they gain through bibliotherapy will lie unused. Each of these skills—taking another's point of view, solving problems systematically, and setting personal goals—emerges gradually and strengthens as children grow in both age and experience.

Role-taking. Stepping into the fictional world of books and film characters is a complex accomplishment for young readers. The early work of Richard Selman (1980) suggests that children younger than five years naively assume that other people see what they see, hear what they hear, know what they know, and will act just as they do. Although they act out different feelings and roles during their make-believe play, these very young children have only a superficial understanding that their characters might act differently if they knew something else or felt differently (Perner, Frith, Leslie, and Leekham 1989; Perner and Wimmer 1985, 1988). Thus, they will need considerable adult help to see connections between the characters' actions and their individuality. By age seven, most children realize that other people see, hear, and think differently than they do, but they still are not very good at guessing what the other person knows and thinks (Moore 1979). As a result, they often cannot predict what the other person is likely to do nor explain why the characters acted as they did. Reading can be a valuable opportunity for these children to peek into another person's mind, even if the mind is fictional. Still, seven-year-olds may not understand how a fictional character is like themselves and may need help in applying the fictional solutions to their own problems. By nine or ten, children have become more adept at guessing what others are thinking and feeling, but they still struggle to understand what someone else intended to accomplish by behaving in a particular way (Shantz 1975). Sophisticated abilities to decipher motivations for behaviors are not clearly established until late adolescence (Leadbeater, Hellner, Allen, and Aber 1989; Selman 1980). In each case, children's hypotheses about another person's behaviors and motivations rely on their understanding of themselves and what they might do in the same situation (Stein and Goldman 1979). Consequently, children's social understanding develops first for scenes familiar to the child and for characters most like the child (Cairns 1986; Selman and Byrne 1974). These will be the easiest characters for them to understand and use as guides.

Problem solving. Child psychologists have broken problem solving into several smaller steps: describing the problem clearly, thinking of more than one solution to the problem, guessing what the consequences of different solutions might be, and choosing the solution that is most likely to work (Spivack, Platt, and Shure 1976). Subsequent research has shown that two kinds of children are successful problem solvers: those who think of more solutions and those who think of higher-quality solutions (Spivack, Platt, and Shure 1976). Both of these skills increase with age. For example, one study showed that seven-year-olds were able to describe half again as many solutions as five-year-olds (Scarr, Weinberg, and Levine 1986). Older children are also more adept at thinking of solutions that are more likely to be successful. Bibliotherapy can assist children with both of these tasks, by pointing out solutions to problems that they had not thought of and by showing consequences of different solutions in especially vivid and meaningful ways. However, depending upon their age and experience, children may not readily recognize either the solutions or their consequences without careful adult guidance. Developmental research suggests that young children will be far more dependent upon that adult guidance than adolescents.

Goal setting. Recognizing problems and seeing solutions will be of little value to young readers unless they also translate their insight into actions that move them closer to their personal goals. An essential first step is seeing the causal link between goals and the actions taken to reach them. By age four, many children begin to see the plan of actions illustrated in a series of pictures, if adults help, and they can often figure out the purpose of a character's actions (Trabasso, Stein, Rodkin, Park, and Baughn 1992). By the age of five, most children can link goals to a story's series of actions. Still, five-year-olds need help in clarifying what their personal goals are and in setting personal goals that they are likely to reach successfully. Adults will have to help them decide what these goals are. A plan of action makes it possible for a child to move toward a goal one small step at a time, but children as old as seven may not realize that these small steps really do move them closer to the larger goal, so they often give up prematurely. They need on-going help from adults, in the form of praise for incremental improvements in performance and to aid in seeing the connection between each day's improvement and their ultimate goals (Woolfolk 1990). It is not until the age of eleven or twelve that children begin to set personal goals that are realistic, clear, and effective. Even then, they are elated when successful, devastated by failure, and stressed by competition; thus, they continue to need adult assistance in managing the emotional turmoil of difficult personal goals (Nicholls and Miller 1984; Stipek, Recchia, and McClintic 1992).

Summary. Programs of bibliotherapy that are designed for very young children must accommodate that age group's very hesitant social understanding and self-management. Those designed for adolescents can assume that older children are more perceptive and more independent in their applications of literary examples and ideas. In between, adults must carefully match their efforts to the child's emerging social understanding, providing no more help than is necessary but enough assistance to assure the child's ultimate success in applying the examples and ideas gleaned from books.

WHO IS QUALIFIED TO
CONDUCT BIBLIOTHERAPY

As interest in bibliotherapy has grown, so has the dispute over which professionals are qualified to engage in the practice. Those who suggest that bibliotherapy be provided by youth librarians or school library media specialists cite the premise, as discussed by Porte (1987), that reading—especially reading good books—helps the reader cope with life. Others argue that only credentialed mental health professionals should act as bibliotherapists. Those who would involve teachers, librarians, and other child-support professionals explain that talking with children about their feelings, hopes, and dreams is a natural part of being a supportive adult. As Bernstein (1989, 165) says, "Some critics feel that bibliotherapy should only be undertaken by those well versed in psychodynamics, neurosis, and psychotherapy. Others, and I concur, feel it can be and is safely undertaken by those with less sophisticated expertise in human nature: teachers, librarians, doctors, lawyers, parents, and others." Sullivan (1987, 874), speaking specifically about classroom teachers, would agree. "Teachers are not therapists, yet most with whom I have talked find a need to deal with the concerns of today's troubled society. . . . Since she spends more time with these youngsters than any other adult, [one fourth-grade teacher] believes that she can help them work through some of their problems." Lack (1985, 28) explains, "Because group reading and discussion are book-centered, such activities seem as appropriate an activity to the library as story hours are for children."

Spache (1978, 245), too, advocates a broad approach to bibliotherapy qualifications. After acknowledging several sources that recommend bibliotherapy only in situations of serious maladjustment, and treatment only by a trained physician or librarian, he states,

> Such sources are obviously too impressed with the connotations of "therapy," ignoring the fact that almost any type of contact between a child and teacher has effects upon the child's personal and social development. We cannot afford to wait until the pupil's maladjustment reaches serious proportions before attempting to ameliorate it in the classroom. Nor can we expect physicians to have the time or training to direct the bibliotherapeutic efforts of teachers. As for librarians, we would welcome their participation in such efforts, but see no reason to believe that they are better trained in child development or mental hygiene than the average classroom teacher.

Those who would restrict the practice of bibliotherapy caution librarians and teachers about their lack of training in therapeutic skills. For example, Smith (1989, 246) says, "Librarians must be cautioned about the danger of crossing the line between being helpful and venturing into the morass of deep emotional problems." Hynes (1987, 167) states, "It seems important to create a constituency among librarians to urge that librarian/bibliotherapists need to acquire additional professional training." Hendrickson (1988, 41) advises caution: "It must be stressed that such therapy with elementary school children does not take place simply through the reading of a book or story. . . . [T]eachers and librarians are not trained therapists, so care should be taken when attempting to interpret hidden messages." Chatton (1988, 335) also strongly opposes the involvement of librarians in bibliotherapy. She explains,

With little background in therapeutic technique they make the mistake of thrusting a novel about a particular problem at a child who is suffering with the hope that the child will read it and feel better. In fact the exact circumstances of the problem and the response to a reading experience can differ so significantly from child to child that this kind of offhand therapy can do more harm than good.

In the absence of any evidence to resolve the dispute, Pardeck and Pardeck (1986, 3) very sensibly suggest that the level of training depends upon the kind of bibliotherapy being practiced. "[T]he helping person need not have advanced clinical skills. Applying bibliotherapy mainly at the identification and projection stage can be very useful as an approach for assisting children or clients with minor adjustment problems and in particular, for helping children deal with developmental growth." Following their example, we see no need to restrict the practice of developmental bibliotherapy, in which book discussions address typical problems in well-adjusted children and adolescents. At the same time, there appears to be good reason to caution well-intentioned professionals about engaging in clinical bibliotherapy unless they have adequate training in the child and adolescent mental health conditions that such therapy addresses.

What problems are posed by unqualified bibliotherapists? Four essential cautions have been detailed. First, the too-casual prescription of books to children with serious problems can backfire (Chatton 1988). In the same way that a garden hose cannot extinguish a forest fire, fictional characters' simplistic solutions may be insufficient for the child's real-life problem. Or the child may lack the skill or knowledge to use a book's solutions successfully. Whatever the reason, failure can leave the child discouraged and less willing to try again. To make such failures less likely, mental health professionals will carefully assess the extent of a child's problem and the circumstances surrounding it prior to beginning bibliotherapy, and will help the child adjust the book's solutions to be more successful.

Second, a fictional plot that resonates too closely with a child's own painful memories and experiences can be traumatic. Readers have had intense emotional reactions or painful flashbacks that caused them to abandon their attempts to face their problems and left them reluctant to try again (Halliday 1991). Mental health professionals will be alert to the signs of such distress, so that they can stop the activity before the distress becomes detrimental and can teach the child strategies to recognize and deal with the emotional impact.

Third, a fictional plot may lead children to expect unrealistic outcomes for their problems. Fictional characters' dilemmas are usually resolved by the end of the book, but real-life dilemmas seldom conclude so neatly. If a book's circumstances are too different from the children's own, or if children are too young to recognize the differences, it may be difficult for them to accept the compromises that represent their own actual success.

Fourth, the bibliotherapy may simply be ineffective. Without the systematic monitoring and follow-up that mental health professionals provide, children may never try out the understanding they gain from books. They may never create a plan of action, may not get around to trying out the different solutions, or may stop working toward their goals long before they accomplish them. When the problems children face are typical developmental struggles, we can assume that they will find the assistance they need with other people or places. However, when the difficulties they face are extraordinary and health-threatening, the ineffectiveness of unqualified therapeutic services can be tragic.

Unless practicing in collaboration with a mental health professional, responsible media specialists, librarians, and teachers will restrict their practice of bibliotherapy to typical developmental issues and to children without identified emotional disorders. Nevertheless, a dilemma remains. Chapter 3 explains that as many as one-fifth of all school-aged children struggle with a diagnosable psychological disorder, but only one out of twenty actually receives mental health services (Doll 1996). Even bibliotherapists who restrict their activities will find themselves confronted, from time to time, with a child who needs more skilled child therapy than they are prepared to provide. So that these young people can be identified early, chapter 3 provides the reader with assistance in recognizing such children and chapter 6 provides additional guidance to lay practitioners in recognizing serious emotional distress.

Alternatively, some writers suggest collaborative activities among media specialists, librarians, and mental health professionals who wish to conduct bibliotherapy, taking advantage of and building upon the unique skills of each. For example, Hart (1987–1988, 56) says,

> Jewish children's librarians working in synagogues and schools can have special impact as book consultants for bibliotherapy. As a first step, they can build book collections including titles that address life's problems. They can inform teachers, counselors, psychologists, and rabbis of particular books that deal sensitively and effectively with these problems. They can advocate the use of books as tools in the process of therapy. Finally, they can learn to lead discussion groups in concert with a trained therapist.

In addressing school counselors, Gladding and Gladding (1991, 9) said that "librarians and English teachers are usually willing and able to recommend specific books for certain children or problems. . . . Finally, there is always the possibility that the counselor can solicit the services of the school librarian in finding materials on certain subjects and even enlist him or her as an ally in the biblioguidance process." Discussing the use of juvenile fiction with stepfamilies, in an article for counselors, Coleman and Ganong (1990, 329) wrote, "Librarians can also provide information about the contents and literary quality of stepfamily books."

We too suggest that professionals collaborate to bring literature's therapeutic insight to children's attention. Collaboration takes advantage of the special talents offered by each profession and makes it possible for a bibliotherapist to act responsibly and safely in the face of unexpected problems or reactions of young readers. With the mentoring activities that occur between trained professionals—be they librarians, media specialists, teachers, or mental health workers—bibliotherapy can become an appropriate activity for all of these professionals.

EFFECTIVENESS OF BIBLIOTHERAPY

Among media specialists and librarians, there is almost universal acceptance of the idea that bibliotherapy is worthwhile. As Hipple, Yarbrough, and Kaplan (1984, 142) state, "[F]ew practitioners in the helping professions deny that reading problem-centered fiction has considerable value for some people in some setting[s]." However, mental health professionals frequently argue that the evidence supporting bibliotherapy is primarily anecdotal, and so is scientifically unconvincing (Lenkowsky 1987). Pardeck and Pardeck (1986) reviewed thirty-seven studies conducted between 1954 and 1978; because more of these studies documented positive rather than negative results, the authors concluded that bibliotherapy was relatively effective in enhancing assertiveness, attitude change, behavioral change, and self-development, and as a therapeutic technique. Subsequently, Lenkowsky (1987) reviewed many of these same studies and more, but with careful attention to the experimental procedures used. He concluded that, as a body, studies of bibliotherapy were often experimentally flawed, demonstrated conflicting results, and failed to document systematic effects that would justify calling bibliotherapy a legitimate child therapy.

Four experimental issues must be resolved for the evidence supporting the use of bibliotherapy to be convincing. First, results of different studies frequently conflict with one another, with as many studies showing evidence of improvement in young readers subsequent to bibliotherapy programs as studies showing no improvement (Lenkowsky 1987; Stevens and Pfost 1982). Consequently, neither forces favoring nor those disputing the effectiveness of bibliotherapy can claim clear support for their position. It is possible that new studies might demonstrate the reasons why certain bibliotherapy programs were not successful and others were, simultaneously resolving the disagreements in bibliotherapy research and providing useful information about planning successful programs.

Second, results of several studies suggest that, even if successful, the results of bibliotherapy are short-lived (Spevak and Richards 1980; Warner 1980). Unless improvements in social competence or social problem solving are durable, bibliotherapy programs will not be useful strategies for meeting most of the purposes used to justify them.

Third, some studies suggest that bibliotherapy is effective only when used in combination with other therapeutic strategies (Kohutek 1983; Walker and Healy 1980). This is not so serious an indictment of bibliotherapeutic strategies, as combinations of therapeutic strategies that include literature or film might still be more effective than those without. For example, therapeutic programs including literature might prove to be more enjoyable and ultimately more motivating.

Finally, numerous reviews of bibliotherapy research have criticized the methods of data collection, experimental design, and data analysis as being incomplete, inconsistent, insubstantial, and unreliable (Lenkowsky 1987; Stevens and Pfost 1982; Warner 1980). Lenkowsky (1987, 128) summarizes this position adeptly when he says, "The absence of systematic, objective, comparative research, however, suggests that while many believe in bibliotherapy and are using it, sufficient substantiated evidence of how it works, why it works, or if it works, is not yet available."

Assistance in resolving this conflict is offered by a line of carefully conducted studies on the impact of self-help books (Rosen 1987; Barrera, Rosen, and Glasgow 1981). In these studies, psychologists have found that self-help manuals are most likely to be effective when (1) the therapist carefully identifies the presenting problem before selecting the book; (2) the therapist maintains ongoing contact with clients to ensure that they follow all instructions carefully; and (3) the therapist steps in to correct or adjust the plan when faced with evidence that the original plan is not working (Rosen 1987). Thus, the systematic follow-up and evaluation activities described in clinical bibliotherapy represent the best plan for effective bibliotherapy.

We conclude by quoting from Moody and Limper's (1971, 6) call for more research. "This continuing and varied interest in bibliotherapy and the expansion of therapeutic library services points up the need for gathering quantitative data, and for evaluating the methods and materials currently in use."

SUMMARY

As this review of the literature of bibliotherapy shows, there is wide and continued interest among many different professionals in using books and other materials to help children and young adults. There is no widespread agreement about who should practice bibliotherapy, what it is, and when it is necessary. It is our intent in this book to address these issues and provide practical suggestions about bibliotherapy that can be useful to everyone.

REFERENCES

Anderson, Marcella F. 1992. "Literature in the Pediatric Setting: The Use of Books to Meet the Emotional and Cognitive Needs of Chronically Ill Children." In *Many Faces, Many Voices: Multicultural Literacy Experiences for Youth,* ed. Anthony L. Manna and Carolyn S. Brodie. Fort Atkinson, WI: Highsmith Press, pp. 79–86.

Ashley, L. F. 1987. "Bibliotherapy and Reading Interests: Patterns, Pitfalls, and Predictions." In *A Track to Unknown Water,* ed. Stella Lees. Metuchen, NJ: Scarecrow Press, pp. 209–22.

Barrera, M., Jr., G. M. Rosen, and R. E. Glasgow. 1981. "Rights, Risks, and Responsibilities in the Use of Self-help Psychotherapy." In *Preservation of Clients Rights,* ed. J. T. Hannah, R. Clark, and P. Christians. New York: Free Press, pp. 204–20.

Bernstein, Joanne E. 1989. "Bibliotherapy: How Books Can Help Young Children Cope." In *Children's Literature: Resource for the Classroom,* ed. Masha Kabakow Rudman. Norwood, MA: Christopher-Gordon Publishing, pp. 159–73.

Bump, Jerome. 1990. "Innovative Bibliotherapy Approaches to Substance Abuse Education." *The Arts in Psychotherapy* 17: 355–62.

Cairns, R. B. 1986. "A Contemporary Perspective on Social Development. In *Children's Social Behavior: Development, Assessment and Modification,* ed. P. S. Strain, M. J. Guralnick, and H. M. Walker. Orlando, FL: Academic Press, pp. 3–91.

Chatton, Barbara. 1988. "Apply with Caution: Bibliotherapy in the Library." *Journal of Youth Services in Libraries* (Spring): 334–38.

Cianciolo, P. J. 1965. "Children's Literature Can Affect Coping Behavior." *Personnel and Guidance Journal* 43: 897–905.

Coleman, Marilyn, and Lawrence H. Ganong. 1990. "The Uses of Juvenile Fiction and Self-help Books with Stepfamilies." *Journal of Counseling and Development* (January/February): 327–31.

Colville, Bruce. 1990. "Magic Mirrors." *Bookmark* (Fall): 35–36.

Doll, B. 1996. "Prevalence of Psychiatric Disorders in Children and Youth: An Agenda for Advocacy by School Psychology." *School Psychology Quarterly* 11: 1–27.

Dreyer, Sharon Spredemann. 1989. *The Bookfinder: Volume 4.* Circle Pines, MN: American Guidance Services.

Frasier, M., and C. McCannon. 1981. "Using Bibliotherapy with Gifted Children." *Gifted Child Quarterly* 25: 81–84.

Gladding, Samual T., and Claire Gladding. 1991. "The ABCs of Bibliotherapy for School Counselors." *School Counselor* (September): 7–13.

Good, Carter. 1966. *Dictionary of Education.* New York: McGraw-Hill.

Gubert, Betty K. 1993. "Sadie Peterson Delaney: Pioneer Bibliotherapist." *American Libraries* (February): 124–30.

Halliday, G. 1991. "Psychological Self-help Books—How Dangerous Are They?" *Psychotherapy* 28(4): 678–80.

Halsted, J. 1988. *Guiding Gifted Readers.* Columbus, OH: Ohio Psychology Publishing.

Hart, Merrily F. 1987–1988. "Bibliotherapy and the Judaica Children's Librarian." *Judaica Librarianship* (Fall/Winter): 56–59.

Hébert, Thomas P. 1991. "Meeting the Affective Needs of Bright Boys Through Bibliotherapy." *Roeper Review* (Roeper City and Country School, MI) 13(4): 207–12.

Hendrickson, Linda B. 1988. "The 'Right' Book for the Child in Distress." *School Library Journal* (April): 40–41.

Hipple, Theodore W., Jane H. Yarbrough, and Jeffrey S. Kaplan. 1984. "Twenty Adolescent Novels (and More) That Counselors Should Know About." *School Counselor* (November): 142–48.

Hynes, Arleen McCarty. 1987. "Bibliotherapy—The Interactive Process." *Catholic Library World* (January/February): 167–70.

———. 1990. "Possibilities for Biblio/Poetry Therapy Services in Libraries." *Catholic Library World* (May/June): 264–67.

Jeon, Kyung-Won. 1992. "Bibliotherapy for Gifted Children." *Gifted Child Today* (November/December): 16–19.

Kohutek, K. J. 1983. "Bibliotherapy Within a Correctional Setting." *Journal of Clinical Psychology* 39(6): 920–24.

Lack, Clara Richardson. 1985. "Can Bibliotherapy Go Public?" *Collection Building* (Spring): 27–32.

Leadbeater, B. J., I. Hellner, J. P. Allen, and J. L. Aber. 1989. "Assessment of Interpersonal Negotiation Strategies in Youth Engaged in Problem Behaviors." *Developmental Psychology* 25: 465–72.

Lenkowsky, Ronald S. 1987. "Bibliotherapy: A Review and Analysis of the Literature." *Journal of Special Education* 21(2): 123–32.

Moody, Mildred T., and Hilda K. Limper. 1971. *Bibliotherapy: Methods and Materials.* Chicago: American Library Association.

Moore, S. G. 1979. "Social Cognition: Knowing About Others." *Young Children* 34: 54–61.

Nicholls, J. G., and A. Miller. 1984. "Conceptions of Ability and Achievement Motivation." In *Research on Motivation in Education, Vol. 1: Student Motivation,* ed. R. Ames and C. Ames. New York: Academic Press, pp. 39–73.

Pardeck, Jean A., and John T. Pardeck. 1984a. "An Overview of the Bibliotherapeutic Treatment Approach: Implications for Clinical Social Work Practice." *Family Therapy* 11(3): 241–52.

———. 1984b. *Young People with Problems: A Guide to Bibliotherapy.* Westport, CT: Greenwood Press.

————, comps. 1986. "Books for Early Childhood: A Developmental Perspective." In *Bibliographies and Indexes in Psychology, Number 3*. New York: Greenwood Press.

Pardeck, John T. 1989a. "Bibliotherapy and the Blended Family." *Family Therapy* 16(3): 215–26.

————. 1989b. "Children's Literature and Adoption." *Child Psychiatry Quarterly* 22: 115–23.

————. 1990a. "Children's Literature and Foster Care." *Family Therapy* 17(1): 61–65.

———— 1990b. "Using Bibliotherapy in Clinical Practice with Children." *Psychological Reports* 67: 1043–49.

————. 1994. "Using Literature to Help Adolescents Cope with Problems." *Adolescence* (Summer): 421–27.

Perner, J., U. Frith, A. M. Leslie, and S. Leekham. 1989. "Exploration of the Autistic Child's Theory of Mind: Knowledge, Belief, and Communication." *Child Development* 60: 421–27.

Perner, J., and H. Wimmer. 1985. "John Thinks That Mary Thinks That . . . Attribution of Second-Order Beliefs by 5- to 10-Year-Old Children." *Journal of Experimental Child Psychology* 39: 437–71.

————. 1988. "Misinformation and Unexpected Change: Testing the Development of Epistemic-State Attribution." *Psychological Research* 50: 191–97.

Porte, Barbara Ann. 1987. "Literature: A Primary Life-Support System." *School Library Journal* (December): 41–42.

Rosen, G. M. 1987. "Self-help Treatment Books and the Commercialization of Psychotherapy." *American Psychologist* 42: 46–51.

Scarr, S., R. A. Weinberg, and A. Levine. 1986. *Understanding Development.* San Diego, CA: Harcourt Brace Jovanovich.

Selman, R. L. 1980. *The Growth of Interpersonal Understanding.* New York: Academic Press.

Selman, R. L., and D. F. Byrne. 1974. "A Structural-developmental Analysis of Levels of Role Taking in Middle Childhood." *Child Development* 45: 803–6.

Shantz, C. U. 1975. "The Development of Social Cognition." In *Review of Child Development Research* 5, ed. E. M. Hetherlington. Chicago: University of Chicago Press.

Smith, Alice. 1989. "Will the Real Bibliotherapist Please Stand Up?" *Journal of Youth Services in Libraries* (Spring): 241–49.

Spache, George D. 1978. "Using Books to Help Solve Children's Problems." *Bibliotherapy Sourcebook,* ed. Rhea Joyce Rubin. Phoenix, AZ: Oryx Press, pp. 240–50.

Spevak, P. A., and C. S. Richards. 1980. "Enhancing the Durability of Treatment Effects: Maintenance Strategies in the Treatment of Nailbiting." *Cognitive Therapy and Research* 4(2): 251–58.

Spivack, G., V. V. Platt, and M. B. Shure. 1976. *The Problem-solving Approach to Adjustment.* San Francisco: Jossey-Bass.

Stein, N. L., and S. Goldman. 1979. "Children's Knowledge About Social Situations: From Causes to Consequences." *Technical Report #147 of the Center for the Study of Teaching.* Champaign: University of Illinois at Urbana Champaign.

Stevens, M. J., and K. S. Pfost. 1982. "Bibliotherapy: Medicine for the 80's." *Psychology: A Quarterly Journal of Human Behavior* 19(4): 21–25.

Stipek, D., S. Recchia, and S. McClintic. 1992. "Self-evaluation in Young Children." *Monograph of the Society for Research in Child Development.* Series 226, Vol. 57, No. 1. Chicago: Society for Research in Child Development/University of Chicago Press.

Sullivan, Joanna. 1987. "Read Aloud Sessions: Tackling Sensitive Issues Through Literature." *Reading Teacher* (May): 874–78.

Trabasso, T., N. Stein, P. Rodkin, M. Park, and C. Baughn. 1992. "Knowledge of Goals and Plans in the On-line Narration of Events." *Cognitive Development* 7: 133–70.

Walker, L. S., and M. Healy. 1980. "Psychological Treatment of a Burned Child." *Journal of Pediatric Psychology* 5(4): 395–404.

Warner, L. 1980. "An Autistic Child and Books." *School Library Journal* 27(2): 107–11.

Woolfolk, A. E. 1990. *Educational Psychology,* 4th ed. Englewood Cliffs, NJ: Prentice Hall.

3 Mental Health Needs of Children and Adolescents

Walk into any elementary school classroom. If there are twenty-five children in the room, national averages tell us that five of those children probably meet the psychiatric criteria for one or more mental illnesses (Brandenberg, Friedman, and Silver 1990; Doll 1996). If the averages hold, at least four of the five are struggling with excessive rates of anxiety. Another one or two children are likely to have attention deficit disorder and are probably hyperactive as well. One of the children might have a conduct disorder, a pattern of noncompliance that also includes serious violations of social rules or laws. If you were to walk into the next classroom, there would probably be another five children with mental illnesses, and another five children in the next room, and so on.

If you entered a high school classroom, the pattern would change somewhat. You would still find at least five students with diagnosable psychiatric disorders, but averages suggest that one of them would probably be clinically depressed. Two or three of the students are likely to be actively contemplating suicide (Reynolds and Mazza 1994). Three students probably have all the symptoms of conduct disorder, perhaps with more persistent and severe symptoms than were evident in the elementary classrooms. One of the young women in the class may be struggling with an eating disorder (Lewinsohn et al. 1993). It is likely that two or three students are using substances to the point of abuse (Murray, Perry, O'Connell, and Schmid 1987). And again, four of the students are likely to be struggling with excessive rates of anxiety.

Who is treating these mental health needs? In all too many cases, no one. National figures document that only 5 percent of school-aged children and youth are currently receiving mental health services, with private or public funding (Knitzer 1982, 1993; Pothier 1988). Other records show that approximately 1 percent of children are served through school districts' special education programs for students with emotional disabilities (Fitzgerald 1987). Presumably, some of those are the same children receiving community services. Even if that were not the case, it is clear that 14 percent of school-aged children and youth have significant mental health needs and are *not* receiving community-based mental health services.

This gap defines the special challenge faced by those who would use books as therapy; librarians and media specialists have no way of knowing which of the children standing before them is struggling with a serious mental health condition, but chances are very good that those who are will not be receiving professional care. Even very caring adults can unwittingly exacerbate a child's emotional distress if they are naive about the impact and expression of a child's emotional disorder. This danger leads many mental health professionals to express serious misgivings about the practice of bibliotherapy by persons without mental health training.

What is to be done? It is unlikely that funds to pay for pediatric mental health services will triple or quadruple in the near future, and so it is not possible to wait to serve these children until adequate mental health support is available. Nor is it sound to withhold the healing power of books from those children most in need of comfort. In chapter 8, we pose another alternative—that of a partnership between media specialists and mental health professionals for the express purpose of using books to assuage the social and emotional distress of children and adolescents.

Every adult involved in raising the community's children, knowingly or unknowingly, becomes jointly responsible for their mental health. To better prepare you for this task, the remainder of this chapter describes the common mental health needs of school-aged children and youth. Chapter 6 lists warning signs that tell when a child's need for therapeutic support has become urgent.

CHILDREN'S MENTAL HEALTH NEEDS

Specialists describe the mental health needs of children and adolescents in three different ways: through a description of developmentally typical problems of children and youth; by identifying the risk factors that predict probable development of a psychiatric disorder; and by traditional diagnosis of the psychiatric disorders of children and youth. Each of these methods describes a somewhat different group of children as being at risk, defines the needs of those children in different ways, and prescribes different kinds of support and assistance.

Developmentally Typical Psychosocial Problems

Childhood is an emotionally tumultuous time. Children struggle with their friendships, in part because they have not yet mastered the ability to understand others' points of view and to negotiate effective compromises when conflicts occur

(Doll, 1996). They struggle with their emotionality because they lack the words they need to label and talk about feelings and because they lack the experiences necessary for moderating the impact that feelings have on their behavior (Wittmer, Doll, and Strain, in press). They struggle with self-control and are still learning to direct their behaviors in ways that serve their future goals (Doll, Sands, Wehmeyer, and Palmer, 1996). Indeed, it is not the occurrence of problems that sets one child apart from another—all children struggle as part of growing up. However, children with more limited success in solving their developmental problems may be at risk for high levels of personal distress and may be less successful in meeting their adult responsibilities, including work, family, and community. Mental health professionals who work with developmentally typical problems do so not with the intent of labeling and identifying children, but to direct adult assistance so that it will most benefit the child.

An early but prominent effort to describe the developmentally typical problems of children and youth was that of Erik Erikson (1963). He described developmental tasks that should be mastered at each age if a child is to develop in a wholesome and adjusted way. For example, Erikson suggested that very young children are struggling to trust that adults will be a consistent and predictable source of care and nurturance. Failing to learn this makes it very difficult for the child to enter into trusting relationships with others in the future. Toddlers are working to achieve a self-restraint that will let them make their own decisions while still complying with social regulations. If they are unable to do this, their opportunities to become self-determined adults are reduced. Three- through six-year-olds are becoming competitive and ambitious and must learn to reconcile their own needs with those of others. Failure to do so will limit their ability to participate in cooperative, community-enhancing ventures. Elementary schoolchildren are learning to overcome their fears of failure when they attempt new skills and acquire ever-increasing amounts of knowledge. Those who are unable to do so can fall into self-defeating patterns of giving up or berating themselves, patterns that limit their success and confidence in new endeavors. Adolescents are struggling to reconcile their individuality with their need to be part of a peer group. If they are not able to create a strong self-identity, they could be easily swayed by group opinions and goals. Erikson suggested that even older children return, periodically, to revisit the struggles that they earlier mastered; consequently, these developmental struggles become enduring themes that attract children's interest and dominate their social understanding.

More recently, Thomas Achenbach (1991) has worked to define the typical behavior problems that emerge at different ages. Working from an extensive list of the behavior problems that caretakers describe in children, he asked parents and teachers to select those that were "somewhat like" and "most like" their child. From their responses, he determined the proportion of children described as having a particular problem across the ages. Thus, Achenbach's results show that being overactive and fidgety is typical among 80 percent of six- and seven-year-olds but only 30 percent of sixteen-year-olds. Twelve-year-olds are twice as likely to be self-conscious as seven-year-olds. In contrast, arguing, being defiant, and having temper tantrums are most common between the ages of eight and fourteen, as is being teased. Swearing, being tardy, and being truant are more typical of adolescents than younger children. Although each of these problems concerns adults, and is often quite inconvenient for adults to contend with, the fact that these problems are quite prevalent during certain ages suggests that they do not represent developmental disturbances. Still, their expression and successful resolution can be critical to comfortable relationships between children and adults.

The work of both Erikson and Achenbach describes problems that challenge children at different ages. The impact that these problems have on children's lives is not diminished merely because they are developmentally typical. Though normal, they are nevertheless challenging and difficult for the child to master, and can be the origin of painful intrapersonal stress. Thus, one goal of bibliotherapy is to provide children and youth with understanding and assistance that will help them face these challenges and lessen their distress in the immediate present. A second goal is to prevent the problems from persisting into later developmental stages, when the problems would no longer be typical.

Psychosocial Risk

Children and adolescents in crisis are disproportionately drawn from families that are impoverished, overcrowded, and struggling with marital discord, child abuse, and dysfunctional parenting practices (Kolvin, Miller, Fleeting, and Kolvin 1988; Rutter 1988; Sameroff, Seifer, and Zax 1982). Moreover, there is convincing evidence that these five factors predict a variety of maladaptive outcomes for children, including lower IQ, higher rates of mental disorders, and higher rates of criminal behavior. The accumulation of factors heightens risk, so even if children can cope with one or two factors, they are likely to suffer detrimental effects when subjected to three or more factors simultaneously.

Unfortunately, these identified risk factors are currently all too common among children and youth. Child poverty rates hover around 25 percent and are expected to increase in the coming decade (Center for the Study of Social Policy 1992). Parental violence against children is rampant, with nearly 11 percent of parents anonymously reporting that they used physically violent discipline against their children in the past year (Gelles and Straus 1987). Marital discord is evidenced by almost 25 percent of students living only with their mothers subsequent to a divorce or when parents never married (U.S. Bureau of the Census 1990). An NIMH study estimated that one of four parents suffered from a mental or addictive disorder during 1992. Thus, significant numbers of children and youth are exposed to the very risk factors most likely to result in lowered intellectual ability, heightened psychiatric distress, or criminal behavior.

Some children are resilient, despite high rates of social risk, because they are able to form effective relationships with adults and peers. Relationships appear to insulate children against the deleterious effects of these risks and provide them with the stamina and social support to achieve competence, despite limiting life situations. Thus, programs that seek to ameliorate risk, including programs of bibliotherapy, attempt to create opportunities for children to interact with and successfully achieve within both peer and cross-age groups. Providing children with an opportunity to meet and discuss books with other children with similar interests can foster relationships that subsequently will support and assist them in times of stress.

Mental Disorders

Mental health specialists divide childhood disorders into internalizing and externalizing disorders. *Internalizing disorders* are those in which a child's inner feelings of distress and tension are excessive. The internalizing child reacts to stressful events by withdrawing into solitude, avoiding difficult situations, and worrying to excess. *Externalizing disorders* are those in which a child's external expressions of distress are excessive. The externalizing child reacts to stressful events by misbehaving, acting aggressively, and disrupting others. In both cases, the children's needs are by-products of their native dispositions and the kind and degree of stresses that exist in their homes and communities. Mental health specialists believe that disorders of this magnitude are debilitating to children and so require skilled mental health services (American Psychiatric Association 1994); nevertheless, many children with these disorders are not currently receiving therapy.

Internalizing Disorders

Anxiety disorders hold the dubious distinction of being one of the most commonly occurring and least commonly treated internalizing disorders among children and adolescents. This may be because only the children have firsthand knowledge of how anxious they are feeling, or because anxious children are likely to be less disruptive and consequently less inconvenient for their adult caregivers; thus, they are not readily referred for services. Interestingly, anxiety-related conditions are among the most common mental illnesses treated among adults, suggesting that once they gain the authority to self-determine when they need help, anxious persons seek assistance at a much higher rate.

Feeling anxious is often described as feeling excessively fearful, but those words are insufficient to capture the experience. Children who are anxious report physical symptoms such as nausea, shortness of breath, sweating or chills, a racing pulse, physical weakness, and uncontrollable shaking. They dwell on thoughts about being out-of-control and worry about disasters that seem to loom nearby, even while they attempt to determine what has occurred to make them anxious. In some cases, when the onset of the anxiety is sudden and unexpected, and the experience is especially intense, the term *panic attack* is used instead. Anxiety can be caused by the situation a child is in, as when a first-grader becomes very anxious upon leaving home for the first time, or can overcome a child apparently without warning. In the latter case, the suspicion is that the cause of the anxiety was biological rather than situational. Certain medications, illicit drugs, and food allergies may have side effects that mimic anxiety attacks.

Because anxiety is "normal," we find it difficult to determine when it is excessive. A large proportion of the mentally healthy public feels overly anxious from time to time; that anxiety may even have interfered with performance or life success. Adults who avoid public speaking, riding on airplanes, climbing to high places, or staying in confined spaces are undoubtedly struggling with anxiety experiences that can be life-impairing. Certain developmental psychologists argue that the degree to which one experiences and reacts to anxious feelings, and the intensity of those feelings, is a temperamental characteristic present at birth, and may even be biologically based and inherited.

To differentiate them from normal fears and anxieties, anxiety disorders are diagnosed only when a child's or adolescent's response to anxiety seriously interferes with his or her life activities and lasts for at least six months. Children's nonadaptive responses to anxiety may take the form of phobias, manifested when they strenuously avoid the object, place, or event that they believe to be causing their anxiety. Such phobias may include avoidance of public places (agoraphobia), being at school (school phobia), speaking in front of others (elective mutism), or taking tests (performance anxiety). Paradoxically, the actual anxiety underlying the phobia may not be visible to an outside observer as long as the child is able to avoid the thing he or she fears. Even if children do not avoid the feared experience, their intense anxiety may still interfere with their performance, as occurs with test anxiety or stage fright. These performance anxieties may be more readily apparent to observers than avoidance behaviors if the physical signs of the anxiety attack are visible—the shaking and the pale face.

The danger of anxiety disorders is that children will work to avoid experiences and places to the point where they cannot live a normal, self-enhancing life. The tragedy of anxiety disorders is that the children will not be able to demonstrate, nor will they be given credit for, competencies they actually have. Without assistance, a child's anxiety disorder may steadily worsen and become ever more disabling.

Obsessive-compulsive disorder (OCD) is a special case of anxiety disorder in which children's or adolescents' minds are invaded by recurrent, unwelcome thoughts or impulses (the obsessions) that cause them to feel extremely anxious. Common obsessions include worries about being unclean, about inadvertently hurting someone, or about needing to keep objects or places in order. Engaging in repetitive, ritualistic actions (the compulsions) lessens the anxiety temporarily. For example, children with obsessive-compulsive disorder may wash their hands until they are chapped and bleeding, perform elaborate rituals when entering a room, or engage in excessive counting, checking, or grooming rituals. Still, the relief gained by performing the rituals is only temporary, and over time the child with OCD experiences the need to repeat these rituals over and over. Because children know that these are strange behaviors and illogical thoughts, they frequently hide their struggle from others, lest they be thought to be crazy. In fact, OCD is such a hidden disorder that it was all but unidentified in young children until recently. Studies have shown that a large proportion of adults with OCD have been struggling with the symptoms since their own childhood; presumably, a few children with OCD might be present in most schools.

If left untreated, the compulsions associated with OCD can come to occupy an inordinate amount of children's time, disturbing their concentration and minimizing their achievements. Moreover, their hidden worries that they are going crazy can be painful and unnecessary. Thus, the danger of OCD is that it will obscure a child's competence and block future achievement.

The term *eating disorders* describes the bizarre eating rituals that certain teenage girls practice in order to manage their weight. Two types of eating disorders are evident: *bulimia,* in which girls become trapped in cycles of bingeing and purging, and *anorexia nervosa*, in which they dangerously restrict their body weight. Though eating disorders are largely a feminine phenomenon, occasional eating disorders are now emerging among males, especially those participating in sports competitions with strict weight limits.

Bulimia is a disorder in which girls alternate between consuming large amounts of food (similar in many respects to the excessive eating that might occur during holiday meals or celebrations) and then purging what they have eaten through induced vomiting, misuse of laxatives, or strenuous exercise. Girls who are bulimic typically feel ashamed of their overeating, are overcritical of their appearance, and work to hide their eating behaviors. Although bulimia is not usually fatal, the physical abuse imposed by repeated purging can have serious health consequences for these girls.

Anorexia nervosa is the more critical eating disorder, in which the girls control food intake to the point where their weight drops to 85 percent or less of healthy weight. In most cases, a girl who is anorexic will control her weight through gross restrictions on the amount that she eats. In addition, these girls struggle with a very distorted image of their body weight or shape, and may battle with symptoms of depression as a by-product of the starvation to which they subject their bodies. Because of their failure to maintain normal body weight, anorexia nervosa is fatal for up to 10 percent of those who suffer from it (American Psychiatric Association 1994).

Both bulimia and anorexia nervosa tend to be hidden disorders. Girls rarely identify themselves as needing assistance, although they may be identified by their parents or by other students if their appearance begins to suggest starvation, if they are caught in the act of purging, or if depressive symptoms begin to emerge. In addition to the physical dangers associated with eating disorders, the girls are also at risk for confidence-impairing struggles with poor body image and limited self-esteem.

Depression has been equated in the public's mind with being very sad, but sadness is only one of the symptoms of depression, and it may not be present in all cases. Instead, depression is characterized by a complex combination of emotional, physical, and cognitive symptoms that frequently cause the person to behave in ways that worsen the depression. Although it is relatively uncommon for young children to develop full clinical depression, adolescents appear to be prone to depression in somewhat larger numbers than adults.

The emotional experience of depression is difficult to describe to people who have not experienced it. Some depressed children report the expected feelings of sadness and despair, but others describe a feeling of emotional emptiness instead of sadness, and report that the emptiness is far more frightening. In addition, depression typically saps youths' ability to find pleasure, even in experiences or events that they had previously enjoyed. In many cases, the children and adolescents become easily irritated or unpredictably angry when depressed, a visible sign of their inner emotional turbulence.

Depression is also characterized by discouraging thoughts about oneself and one's accomplishments. While depressed, it is difficult for adolescents to recognize their personal triumphs or successes. Instead, they become preoccupied with their shortcomings, are quick to blame themselves for any problems that occur, and become locked into pessimistic ruminations about the hopelessness of ever reaching their goals and aspirations. Most depressed persons describe difficulty concentrating, especially in the face of distractions. They tend to put off making decisions and procrastinate when pressed to take action. In some, but not all, cases, a person who is depressed will contemplate suicide or other forms of self-injury.

When depression is severe, the suffering children and adolescents may withdraw into a cocoon of social isolation. They avoid friends and acquaintances who were previously central to their daily lives, and instead spend large portions of the day sitting alone and doing very little. Their inactivity may intensify to the point that their school work suffers, as does their satisfaction from work or family responsibilities. Their self-enforced isolation and inactivity can be especially frustrating for friends and family members who recognize the trouble the children are in and see how their behavior is feeding it.

The physical experience of depression is one of oppressive fatigue. Children who are depressed often move more slowly and with obvious exhaustion, and their posture may drag as if to act out the emotional weight they carry. In some cases, this fatigue is understandable, because of their pervasive insomnia, but other children sleep to excess. Disruptions in appetite and eating are also common, and many depressed youth revert to a diet of caffeinated soft drinks and little else. Other physical complaints include nausea, headaches, or vague complaints of feeling dizzy or unwell. Depression can occur in conjunction with anxiety disorders, and some children abuse substances in an apparent attempt to self-medicate their own depression.

Although less common, bouts of depression in adolescents can be interspersed with periods of euphoria. These manic episodes are marked by uncharacteristic enthusiasm, uncritical self-confidence, and boundless energy. The hidden danger of manic episodes is the imprudent and impulsive decisions that adolescents make under their influence—decisions to engage in indiscriminate and excessive sexual behaviors, dangerous driving behaviors, shopping to the point of bankruptcy, or gambling. Other, less dangerous excesses include nonstop talking, avoiding sleep, and easy irritability. Moreover, the manic episode is almost always followed by a crashing depression that is overwhelming in its contrast with the euphoria.

One of the most striking dangers of depression is that it will go unrecognized. Left untreated, depression can linger for several years, sapping children's competence and limiting their engagement in developmental tasks of schooling and socializing. Not only would we regret leaving a child with the psychological pain of depression, but we also know that children who are locked into a cycle of emotional despair and biological fatigue are unlikely to persist in the face of minor obstacles, and instead give up many potential opportunities. School achievements and other tasks will be significantly lower than a child's expected capabilities.

Suicide and suicidal behaviors. As many as 11 percent of the students in a high school are actively contemplating suicide, and studies suggest that two-thirds of these are students with depression. The range of suicidal behaviors in which students engage extends from simple thoughts of death and dying to actual suicide attempts. For practical purposes, we divide this range into three stages.

In the first stage of *ideation,* adolescents actively think about death and dying and may wish that they had never been born. They may construct elaborate fantasies about what would happen after their deaths—fantasies in which others would realize how valuable they had been, or would be punished by guilt. The ideation phase may progress to the point where students make actual plans for a suicide attempt. These plans can be ranked according to their lethality by the following factors: the likelihood that children would die using that method, how likely they are to be interrupted or rescued, and how possible it is for them to change their minds after starting the attempt.

Some youths move from ideating into the second, *intent,* stage when they begin to act out the early stages of their suicidal plans. They may write notes, make a will, or begin to arrange their personal affairs in preparation for death. In some cases, they engage in minor self-destructive actions, such as cutting themselves or practicing high-risk, dangerous behaviors. They may make subtle or overt threats of suicide to others.

In the third stage, *attempt,* young people make an actual suicide attempt. If the attempt is unlikely to succeed, either because their choice of method was unlikely to be lethal or because they made the attempt in a way that was likely to be interrupted, the attempt may be called a *pseudo-attempt.* In either case, adolescents who have made one suicide attempt are at serious risk of making another.

The proportion of students actually reaching the attempt stage is surprisingly high, representing 3.5 percent of the high-school-age population. Imprecise records make it difficult to determine the prevalence of successful suicides in young adults, but experts estimate a prevalence of 1 death by suicide for every 5,000 to 10,000 adolescents (Cheifetz, Posener, leHaye, Zajdman, and Benierakis 1987; Centers for Disease Control 1987). Moreover, attempts become more prevalent in schools and communities where there has been a recent successful suicide, especially if that suicide is well publicized and if there are striking memorials to the student who died. Given the large numbers of peers who are also contemplating suicide, any dramatic suicide attempt can prod peers to do likewise, leading to the increasingly common phenomenon of cluster suicide. Completed suicides send shock waves through the friends and acquaintances of the deceased youth, and require carefully planned suicide response programs to prevent subsequent "copycat" deaths.

Externalizing Disorders

Attention deficit/hyperactivity disorder (ADHD) is one of the most controversial disorders of childhood. The researchers and clinicians who specialize in its identification and treatment disagree about its prevalence and the principal symptoms that define it. Even its official title has changed twice in the past fifteen years. The child with ADHD behaves in ways that are thoughtless, frequently disruptive, and often in violation of social rules and conventions. More specifically, the disorder is characterized by three clusters of symptoms: impulsivity, inattention, and hyperactivity.

Impulsivity most often marks the difference between children with ADHD and typical children. Children with ADHD answer quickly, without waiting for instructions to be completed or questions to be stated, and consequently they make innumerable careless mistakes. They engage in frequent and unnecessary risk taking without considering the potentially negative or even dangerous consequences of their actions. When required to wait, they tend to badger adults or blurt out thoughtless remarks to peers. Their written work is frequently messy, unorganized, and full of errors.

Paying attention takes effort. To pay attention, a child must disregard irrelevant noises, sights, or thoughts and continue to focus on the task at hand. Children with ADHD can pay attention for very brief periods of time but have difficulty sustaining that effort for longer periods of time. Consequently, they switch frequently from one activity to the next and are frequently uncooperative, especially when the task is repetitive, tedious, or boring.

Many, but not all, children with ADHD show a level of overactivity that is so striking that their diagnosis was once called simply "hyperactivity disorder." When seated, they wiggle restlessly and fidget quietly. At other times, they are unable to stay seated and wander purposelessly back and forth around a room. At still other times, they appear driven and wild, running or flailing seemingly without control. Some children with ADHD talk or chant excessively instead of or in addition to their excessive physical activity.

A child is not identified as having ADHD unless these symptoms are evident in at least two different settings, such as at home, in school, or in public places like stores, churches, or restaurants. Diagnosis is complicated by the fact that the symptoms become minimal or even disappear in some situations—when adults have strict control over behaviors, in unfamiliar situations when the child is uncertain of what will happen, during activities that are especially interesting and provide immediate reinforcement (such as video games), and during one-to-one supervision. Thus, in some situations, a child's ADHD might be all but unnoticeable.

Their frequently irritating behavior makes children with ADHD prime targets for derogatory judgments and comments by peers, teachers, and adult caregivers. Consequently, it is not surprising to find that by middle childhood, most children with attention deficits have self-perceptions that are quite battered and negative. This lowered self-esteem, the principal secondary effect of attention deficits, has become the target of numerous psychological and educational intervention programs that work to enhance the social and emotional adjustment of children with ADHD.

Conduct disorder is an externalizing disorder that has spawned heated ethical debates among schools and other agencies that serve children and adolescents. The persistent noncompliance of children with conduct disorders sorely tries the patience of social agencies, leading some spokespersons to suggest that these very difficult children should simply be excluded from programs and services unless and until they agree to cooperate with the rules of conduct. Opposing viewpoints suggest that both societal and biological causes underlie such a child's noncompliance, and that these children deserve the same commitment to programs and interventions as children with any other psychological disorder.

Not all noncompliant children satisfy the diagnostic criteria for conduct disorders. When a true conduct disorder is present, the child is not only noncompliant, but also is cruelly aggressive to the point that he or she seriously harms other people, damages others' property, is deceitful or steals, and breaks the law (either through persistent truancy or curfew violations in childhood, with more serious offenses occurring in later adolescence). Current prevalence records suggest that between 3 and 5 percent of elementary schoolchildren and between 8 and 13 percent of secondary schoolchildren have conduct disorders this severe. Their ongoing inattention to the consequences of these behaviors, whether to themselves or to other people, leads some persons to suggest that conduct-disordered children are incapable of forming authentic and caring relationships. Although this assertion is controversial, it is true that children with conduct disorders tend to be manipulative, and their relationships are frequently shallow.

When children are noncompliant and difficult, but not deliberately cruel and hurtful, they might be considered to have an oppositional defiant disorder in lieu of a conduct disorder. The aggression of oppositional-defiant children is likely to be verbal rather than physical, and their misbehavior generally stops short of cruelty. Also, though their surface relationships may appear to be difficult and maladaptive, they do have authentic relationships with other people.

Both conduct-disordered and oppositional-defiant children seem to get caught in cycles of aggressive conflict with both adults and children, in which they are reluctant to give in and which are likely to escalate their aggression when thwarted.

Consequently, they have frequently conditioned other people not to challenge them, and they may be distrusted or even avoided by their classmates and peers. Their disrupted relationships, frequent and inflammatory conflicts, and unsatisfactory behavior mean that conduct-disordered children live with constant criticism and disapproval. Thus, it is not surprising to find that some children and adolescents with conduct disorders also show signs of depression or anxiety disorders. These dually diagnosed children are at special risk for adult problems.

SUMMARY

All children and adolescents are challenged by problems as they mature—worries about themselves and their relationships with others, conflicts between what they want and what they can have, and obstacles that stop them from achieving personal goals. The challenges faced by some children loom larger than normal and place them at special risk. An important component of bibliotherapy is understanding how these challenges differ and recognizing the implications these differences hold for a child's competence and independence. This understanding is a particular skill of mental health professionals who specialize in children and adolescents and is the most important contribution that such professionals can make to a bibliotherapy program.

REFERENCES

Achenbach, T. M. 1991. *Manual for the Child Behavior Checklist 4-18 and 1991 Profile.* Burlington: University of Vermont, Department of Psychiatry.

American Psychiatric Association. 1994. *The Diagnostic and Statistical Manual of Mental Disorders.* Washington, DC: Author.

Brandenberg, N. A., R. M. Friedman, and S. E. Silver. 1990. "The Epidemiology of Childhood Psychiatric Disorders: Prevalence Findings from Recent Studies." *Journal of the American Academy of Child and Adolescent Psychiatry* 29: 76–83.

Center for the Study of Social Policy. 1992 (September). *The Challenge of Change: What the 1990 Census Tells Us About Children.* Washington, DC: Author.

Centers for Disease Control. 1987. *Death Rates for 282 Selected Causes of Death in the United States (1979–1985).* Atlanta, GA: Author.

Cheifetz, P. N., J. A. Posener, A. leHaye, M. Zajdman, and C. E. Benierakis. 1987. "An Epidemiologic Study of Adolescent Suicide." *Canadian Journal of Psychiatry* 32: 656–59.

Costello, E. J. 1989. "Child Psychiatric Disorders and Their Correlates: A Primary Care Pediatric Sample." *Journal of the American Academy of Child and Adolescent Psychiatry* 28: 851–55.

Doll, B. 1996. "Children Without Friends: Implications for Practice and Policy." *School Psychology Review* 25: 165–83.

———. 1996. "Prevalence of Psychiatric Disorders in Children and Youth: An Agenda for Advocacy by School Psychology." *School Psychology Quarterly* 11: 1–27.

Doll, B., D. Sands, M. Wehmeyer, and S. Palmer. 1996. "Promoting the Development and Acquisition of Self-determined Behaviors." In *Self-determination Across the Lifespan: Theory and Practice,* ed. D. Sands and M. Wehmeyer. Baltimore, MD: Paul Brookes Publishing.

Erikson, E. H. 1963. *Childhood and Society.* New York: W. W. Norton.

Fitzgerald, I. M. 1987. "Childhood Disability: Prevalence and Incidence." *Marriage and Family Review:* 7–24.

Flament, M. F., A Whitaker, J. Rapoport, M. Davies, C. Zaremba, M. A. Berg, K. Kalikow, W. Sceery, and D. Schaffer. 1988. "Obsessive-Compulsive Disorder in Adolescence: An Epidemiological Study." *Journal of the American Academy of Child and Adolescent Psychiatry* 27: 764–71.

Fleming, J. E., and D. R. Offord. 1990. "Epidemiology of Childhood Depressive Disorders: A Critical Review." *Journal of the American Academy of Child and Adolescent Psychiatry* 29: 571–80.

Gelles, R. J., and M. A. Straus. 1987. "Is Violence Toward Children Increasing? A Comparison of 1975 and 1985 National Survey Rates." *Journal of Interpersonal Violence* 50: 212–22.

Kashani, J. H., and H. Orvaschel. 1990. "A Community Study of Anxiety in Children and Adolescents." *American Journal of Psychiatry* 147: 313–18.

Kashani, J. H., R. K. Rosenberg, and J. C. Reid. 1989. "Developmental Perspectives in Child and Adolescent Depressive Symptoms in a Community Sample." *American Journal of Psychiatry* 146: 871–75.

Knitzer, J. 1982. *Unclaimed Children: The Failure of Public Responsibility to Children and Adolescents in Need of Mental Health Services.* Washington, DC: Children's Defense Fund.

———. 1993. "Children's Mental Health Policy: Challenging the Future." *Journal of Emotional and Behavioral Disorders* 1: 8–16.

Kolvin, I., F. J. W. Miller, M. Fleeting, and P. A. Kolvin. 1988. "Risk and Protective Factors for Offending with Particular Reference to Deprivation." In *Studies of Psychosocial Risk: The Power of Longitudinal Data,* ed. M. Fleeting. New York: Cambridge University Press, pp. 7–95.

Lewinsohn, P. M., H. Hops, R. E. Roberts, J. R. Seeley, and J. A. Andrews. 1993. "Adolescent Psychopathology: Prevalence and Incidence of Depression and Other DSM-III-R Disorders in High School Students." *Journal of Abnormal Psychology* 102: 133–44.

Murray, D. M., C. L. Perry, C. O'Connell, and L. Schmid. 1987. "Seventh-grade Cigarette, Alcohol and Marijuana Use." *International Journal of the Addictions* 22: 357–76.

Offord, D. R., M. H. Boyle, P. Szatmari, N. I. Rae-Grant, P. S. Links, D. T. Cadman, J. A. Byles, J. W. Crawford, H. M. Blum, C. Byrne, H. Thomas, and C. A. Woodward. 1987. "Ontario Child Health Study: Six-month Prevalence of Disorder and Rates of Service Utilization." *Archives of General Psychiatry* 44: 832–36.

Pothier, P. C. 1988. "Child Mental Health Problems and Policy." *Archives of Psychiatric Nursing* 8: 165–69.

Reynolds, W. M., and J. J. Mazza. 1994. "Suicide and Suicidal Behaviors in Children and Adolescents." In *Handbook of Depression in Children and Adolescents,* ed. W. M. Reynolds and H. F. Johnston. New York: Plenum Press, pp. 525–80.

Rutter, M. 1988. "Epidemiological Approaches to Developmental Psychopathology." *Archives of General Psychiatry* 45: 486–95.

Rutter, M., and S. Sandberg. 1985. "Epidemiology of Child Psychiatric Disorder: Methodological Issues and Some Substantive Findings." *Child Psychiatry and Human Development* 15: 209–33.

Sameroff, A. J., R. Seifer, and M. Zax. 1982. "Early Development of Children at Risk for Emotional Disorder." *Monographs for the Society for Research in Child Development* 47.

U.S. Bureau of the Census. 1990 (June). "Studies in Marriage and the Family." *Current Population Reports Series P-23, No. 167*. Washington, DC: U.S. Government Printing Office.

Velez, C. N., J. Johnson, and P. Cohen. 1989. "A Longitudinal Analysis of Selected Risk Factors for Childhood Psychopathology." *Journal of the American Academy of Child and Adolescent Psychiatry* 28: 861–64.

Wittmer, D, B. Doll, and P. Strain. In press. "Assessment of Social/Emotional Development in Young Children." *Journal of Early Intervention*.

4 Skills of the Youth Librarian/ Media Specialist

Public libraries are a part of many communities in the United States, and school library media centers are common at every grade level. But what do professional librarians, information scientists, and media specialists do? Billings (1995, 36) says, "The librarian is educated and trained to deal with the selection, acquisition, organization, service, preservation, and training activities required" to carry out the function of libraries or information centers. Speaking specifically of children's library services, Mae Benne (1991, 2) states: "Within the library the children's librarian assumes responsibilities for (1) selecting and maintaining a collection for the appropriate audiences, (2) providing information and reading guidance (advisory) services, and (3) planning and presenting programs."

To acquire the skills to perform this complex, demanding position, youth librarians pursue a graduate degree that includes study of child and adolescent psychology, as well as many other relevant subjects. Furthermore, school media specialists are normally required to have a teaching certificate and classroom experience.

Using this knowledge, the youth librarian selects, purchases, and organizes materials, then helps children and young adults to locate, use, and—it is hoped—enjoy the books, media, and information belonging to the library or media center collection.

This is an ongoing, never-ending, overwhelming, exciting, and enjoyable process. Three elements of the youth librarian's work are especially applicable to bibliotherapy: knowledge of youth materials, reference skills, and experience in reading guidance.

KNOWLEDGE OF YOUTH MATERIALS

Librarians and media specialists are knowledgeable about children's and young adult materials. They read the books, view the videos, and listen to the recordings. More importantly, youth librarians think critically about the content of these materials and work to separate the good from the bad.

The desire to share quality books with youth is not a recent development. In the late 1800s, Caroline Hewins, the children's librarian, "based her conception of library work on a pure love for books; for her this meant careful selection of the best, a selection rooted in an intimate knowledge of children themselves and based on an acquaintance of the so-called best of world literature" (Heins 1982, 249). For years after this, children's librarians felt an obligation to share quality books with children and lead them away from poorer or formulaic writing such as the Nancy Drew and Hardy Boys books. In today's libraries, children's professionals are still concerned with quality materials. MacDonald asserts, "First you purchase the best books you can find and then you sell the books to kids as if you were on a commission and got bonus points for the good stuff" (Genco, MacDonald, and Hearne 1991, 118). At the same time, however, libraries increasingly acknowledge a place for some of the lower-quality materials that many children and young adults enjoy. To this effect, MacDonald admits, "For my whole professional life I have included some representative titles from the popular, high interest, mass media-based genres in collections" (Genco, MacDonald, and Hearne 1991, 115). Even though library and media center collections may now include some popular, lower-quality materials, nevertheless librarians still emphasize the importance of acquiring good materials.

The quest to identify the best materials for children and young adults has led to many discussions and debates about what qualities make a children's book good. Jean Karl (1982, 256), book editor at Atheneum, said, "The truth is that there are many kinds of best." Charlotte Zolotow (1982, 263), children's author and editor for Harper & Row publishers, wrote, "[I]t is exactly what makes a good adult book. All the criteria of good craftsmanship, talent, and quality of writing are the same. But there is one big difference—the voice!—the point of view of the writer . . . that direct, the-emperor-has-no-clothes-place." Madeline L'Engle, award-winning children's author, agreed: "*[H]ow* you write it, the depth of characterization, of syntax, has got to be just as good as a book written to be marketed for adults" (Zolotow 1982, 264).

There has been and continues to be discussion of exactly what constitutes quality in literature. As youth librarians review, analyze, and discuss the strengths and weaknesses of individual titles, they tend to look at character, plot, theme, setting, point of view, style, and tone. In *A Critical Handbook of Children's Literature*, Rebecca Lukens (1995) presents and discusses each of these elements. Information about fictional characters may be revealed by actions, speech, appearance, or comments by other characters or the author. Flat, less developed characters may and probably should be present in most books. For purposes of bibliotherapy, the characters involved in the situation of interest or displaying the pertinent personality traits should be well-rounded principal characters truly important to the story. Furthermore, these characters should display realistic, believable personalities with which children or young adults can identify.

The *plot* of a story is basically the sequence of events that occur. Though the plot may be episodic or continuous, chronological or flashed-back, it is also the vehicle for conveying the conflict of the story. The conflict may be person against self, person against person, person against society, or person against nature. A good author may use literary devices such as suspense or foreshadowing to lead to the climax and denouement, and the end should seem to flow naturally from the events of the story. Too much reliance on coincidence or sentimentality or a lack of conflict weakens the plot. For purposes of bibliotherapy, the plot should be realistic, exciting, and logical, and details about the topic of interest should be accurate. The better the plot is, the easier it will be for children or young adults to make connections between the book or video and their own lives.

According to Lukens (1995, 87), *theme* "in literature is the idea that holds the story together." The theme may be implied or explicitly stated. Rich, well-developed plots and characters often present multiple themes. As with the endings of stories, the theme should emerge naturally from the story and not be blatantly didactic or preachy. For purposes of bibliotherapy, themes in materials used should be compatible with, not contradictory to, the goals and objectives of the sessions.

Setting refers to the time and place in which a story takes place. The setting may be just the backdrop or stage for the story, or the setting itself may be a vital element, such as in stories where the main conflict is person against nature. The setting should be appropriate to the story and drawn well enough that it does not detract from the story events. In selecting titles for bibliotherapy, remember that the issues presented in a story set in a time or place different from the contemporary United States may be less threatening to children or young adults. This may make it easier to promote discussion. However, remember also that it may be easier for children or young adults to identify with or transfer their insights from a story in a familiar setting.

A story may be told in first person by one of its characters. Or the author may choose to speak in the third person, conveying words, thoughts, feelings, and actions of all characters in the past, present, and future. Alternatively, when speaking in the third person, the author may speak about one main character or a few characters and may choose the objective viewpoint, faithfully recording what is seen or heard but omitting any references to thoughts or feelings.

Any of these *points of view* can be appropriate to a particular story or for bibliotherapy, although each may have different results. However, young readers may identify most closely with a first-person narrator. Access to thoughts and feelings of all characters may be somewhat overwhelming and result in a longer story. At the same time, this technique—or a more limited version of it—does provide children and young adults with insight into the thoughts and feelings of several different people. The objective presentation gives an opportunity for discussion of possible motives or thoughts or feelings implied by the reported speech and action.

Style refers to the specific words chosen by the author and the way those words are used together to convey the story. English classes study the multitude of devices available to writers: connotation, imagery, figurative language, hyperbole, understatement, allusion, symbol, and puns. Any or all of these elements of style can be and have been appropriately used in materials for children and young adults. The most important thing to remember is that the style should be accessible to the anticipated audience. Often a direct, readable style is best for young readers.

The last element of quality discussed by Lukens is *tone,* the attitude that the author has toward the subject presented. One hopes that respect and interest in the topic will be communicated to young readers. Humor is also appropriate and often desirable, provided the author laughs with, not at, the audience. Any indication of condescension or didacticism tends to alienate young people. Moreover, a morose or pessimistic tone may lower the reader's own mood and place those who are emotionally vulnerable at risk.

Further criteria are applied to specific genres. For example, once the ground rules are laid, fantasy must follow the logic of its created universe. In historical fiction, the background information should emerge from the story and not intrude like textbook discourses. Informational materials, in contrast, are evaluated by the author's professional qualifications, accuracy, currency, absence of stereotypes, purpose and scope, intended audience, safety instructions, and illustrations, in addition to indices and other organizational aids (Barron and Burely 1984, 62–63).

Some materials in the library or media center are in an audiovisual or electronic format. Although the same criteria apply to the content of these materials as to the content of print materials, additional elements are considered for determining whether the format is appropriate to the content. For example, a librarian must decide if a story dealing with teenage suicide might be more effectively portrayed through a book that allows characters to voice private thoughts or through the words and actions of a video. Overall, regardless of content or format, the youth librarian carefully selects the items that become a part of the library or media center collection.

Such careful evaluation of and knowledge about the quality of the library or media center collection is important to bibliotherapy. Materials selected for use with children or young adults should be realistic in terms of the people, situations, and solutions presented. Quality materials for children and young adults can satisfy these requirements. As MacDonald noted, "What we should look for in the materials we choose is the connecting human element—the relevance of the story or information to our shared humanity" (Genco, MacDonald, and Hearne 1991, 118). Jean Karl (1982, 257) observed, "In a fine work of fiction we are literally seeing a segment of the world—as it is, as it was, as it could be, or as the author wishes it were—through the author's eyes. This does not mean the writer is doing this consciously. Rather the author is writing about something that so involves him that his deep understandings and perceptions are revealed in what he writes." In this way, a strong writer can accurately portray feelings, fears, relationships, or coping strategies in realistic settings. Even if this portrayal is not intentional, good writers are nevertheless observers and recorders of human nature. Such insights reveal the power and the potential of good materials for helping children and young adults. To this effect, librarians and media specialists can assist mental health professionals to identify appropriate materials for bibliotherapeutic use.

Any library or media center houses a collection of materials (books, videos, computer software or CD-ROMs) designed to meet the curricular, informational, or recreational needs of young users. These materials often serve multiple purposes. For example, a book or CD-ROM on arms and armor of the Middle Ages can meet the curricular needs of a history unit. The same title can also meet the recreational needs of a young user interested in role-playing games.

This same phenomenon occurs for materials appropriate for bibliotherapy. The Newbery award is given annually to the author of the best written book published for children in the United States. Winning titles are in almost all children's collections. At least two of those titles could be appropriate for a bibliotherapy session related to death: *Bridge to Terabithia* by Katherine Paterson (1977) and *Missing May* by Cynthia Rylant (1992).

The important point is that all collections of children's or young adult materials have titles that would be appropriate for bibliotherapy. The youth librarian or media specialist has the knowledge and skills to identify those titles and match them to young users.

REFERENCE SERVICES

The youth librarian or media specialist is specifically trained to provide reference services. Moreover, Radford (1989, 3) emphasizes that "the librarian is the human interface between the library user and the information sources." Library professionals recognize that it is not enough merely to collect and organize materials; they also have an obligation to help users—young or old—to locate information or find items that the users want or need. Reference work or reference services comprise those activities and skills librarians and media specialists employ to help bring together the library user and requested information.

The professional literature and research about reference service in libraries is extensive. Fitzgibbons (1986) notes, though, that much more has been written in this area about adult service than about services for children and young adults. One area of reference service that has been investigated and discussed is the types of reference questions asked by children and young adults. These questions are commonly divided into four categories:

- Directional questions, such as "Where is the water fountain?," may or may not be counted as reference questions by a particular researcher or library.

- Ready-reference questions, such as "Who wrote *Charlotte's Web*?," are relatively quick and easy to answer.

- Informational questions, such as "I need information about divorce," require more time and effort, as the librarian or media specialist may need to consult multiple sources.

- Research questions, such as "What causes depression?," require more extensive searching and may produce multiple, contradictory answers (Horning 1994, 11).

Communication is an integral aspect of reference service. Generally, the user will come to or phone the library or media center with a reference question or information need. After the user and the librarian or media specialist interact, the library professional searches for (or helps the user search for) and, it is hoped, locates the information requested. The chances for a successful exchange are increased when the library professional and the user can effectively communicate with each other.

Extensively written about and researched in the library literature, this process is referred to as the *reference interview*. During the interview, practitioners are urged to practice active listening and to ask open questions (i.e., those that disclose information or details) rather than closed questions (i.e., those that require one-word, yes/no types of answers) (Jennerich and Jennerich 1987). An open, nonjudgmental attitude is also considered important. As Sexton (1977, 178) noted, "To want to help and to try to establish a rapport with the young person are the prime requisites of a good interview."

Research has also been conducted on the types of questions that children and adults may ask. Reporting on a study done at the public library in Urbana, Illinois, Harrington (1985, 65) noted, "[A]dults and children tend to ask different kinds of questions. Children tended to ask for assistance of an essentially mechanical nature, such as help in locating items and assistance with the audiovisual materials. Adults tended to ask complex reader's advisory questions, reference questions, and questions concerning library policies and programs."

To answer reference questions effectively, librarians and media specialists use the materials and information resources available in the library or media center. Moreover, the skills of the reference librarian—knowledge of the collections, ability to conduct a reference interview, and a willingness to search for information—are well suited to bibliotherapy.

Because librarians and media specialists work in an environment where children are present, it is customary for these adult professionals to establish a variety of relationships with their young users. Some interactions are short and casual, as when a child or young adult unknown to the librarian asks for help locating or using information or materials. It is difficult in such cases to determine whether information on the topic, such as divorce, is to meet personal or curricular needs.

Some requests for information from young users, who are either unknown or only slightly known to the librarian or media specialist, may lead to longer, more detailed discussions. The longer interaction may reveal whether the need is personal. Such protracted interactions allow the library professional to evaluate the young person's behavior for the warning signs discussed in chapter 6.

Some children or young adults are regular patrons of their public libraries or school library media centers. Some of these youngsters develop personal relationships with their youth librarian. This gives opportunities for the professional librarian to mentor these young people as they go through the normal process of growing up and dealing with the normal problems and questions that arise. It is beneficial for young people to have good, positive adult role models. Also, it is not unusual for librarians and media specialists to recommend and discuss library materials during this mentoring process.

The librarian or media specialist can also use these skills as a "human interface" in collaborative bibliotherapy work. First, the mental health and library professionals can evaluate a situation and determine the appropriate subject content of materials they wish to share with particular young people. Next, the library professional can identify and locate a range of books, videos, and other materials that address the appropriate issues. Finally, these professionals can work together to select specific titles for the children or young adults.

READING GUIDANCE

Reader's guidance, as used here, is an umbrella term encompassing three types of activities: reader's advisory, book discussions, and booktalks. All three can make important contributions to bibliotherapy.

Reader's Advisory

Reader's advisory services to children and young adults are closely related to, and even considered by some to be a subset of, reference services. In *Advocating Access*, a publication of guidelines for youth services in Washington state libraries, the reader's advisory services section states:

> Staff combine their background in child and adolescent development, parent education, reading and literacy, and language development with an in-depth knowledge of youth collections and a general knowledge of all other collections in the library to help children, young adults, parents and other youth-involved adults locate and use library materials. Communication between library staff and users cultivates reading as a viable individual or group activity, as a means of exploring personal interests and meeting educational needs, and as a lifetime pattern for pleasure and personal growth (Washington Library Association, Children's and Young Adult Services 1989, 14).

The child or young adult may ask for a specific book, for a book by a specific author or on a particular subject, or just for a good book to read (Connor 1985). In addition, the youth librarian or media specialist may take the initiative and suggest a title to a child or young adult. As Fasick (1991) notes, this is primarily an individual service, not a group one.

Reader's advisory is a widespread, firmly established part of library service to youth. A survey done during the fall of 1987 found that 88 percent of public libraries in the United States offered reader's advisory service to young adults for independent needs, and 87 percent offered such services to young adults for school needs (U.S. Department of Education 1988, 8). A similar federal survey of public library services to children was conducted in 1988–1989. In this study, 72 percent of the libraries reported availability of reader's advisory services for children (U.S. Department of Education 1990, iii). Furthermore, *Information Power*, the national standards for school library media centers, indicates that school library media specialists should have in-depth knowledge of "techniques for determining individual needs and interests and for matching them with appropriate materials" (American Association of School Librarians and Association for Educational Communications and Technology 1988, 30). Such examples illustrate the extent to which reader's advisory is a commonly accepted and integral part of library work with children and young adults.

The personal, individual attention of a reader's advisory exchange is an ideal opportunity for the professional librarian to mentor the child or young adult. In this regard, a book, video, or recording can be a neutral, nonthreatening starting point for discussion. Often, youths may need a supportive adult to express interest and concern in their problems. As a trained professional, the librarian or media specialist has the skills and integrity to mentor young people in this way.

However, some children or young adults are more deeply troubled. In these cases, the same skills required to successfully carry out reader's advisory—knowledge of materials, knowledge of young people, and the ability to match the two—enable the librarian or media specialist to make valuable contributions to a bibliotherapy team. By pairing the skills of the library professional with those of the mental health professional (see chapter 3), the resulting partnership exploits the skills of both to enhance service to youth.

Book Discussion

Librarians and media specialists also possess valuable skills for and experience in discussing books, videos, and tapes with groups of children and young adults. These discussions can vary from an informal, spontaneous exchange triggered by youth interest and sustained by the librarian's knowledge to a formal, well-planned program. As the library literature indicates, discussion programs have existed for many years in many formats. *Let's Talk About It* is a planner's manual designed to help librarians or media specialists plan, promote, execute, and evaluate a book discussion program (Moores and Rubin 1984).

Youth librarians can use their skills in material selection to identify specific titles for use in group discussion. Short stories or books, videos, or audio recordings may be shared with the entire group prior to discussion. Young people may be asked to read longer books before coming to a session at which the whole group discusses the book, film, or recording. Questions or topics for discussion are prepared in advance, based on the youth librarian's familiarity with the materials. This preparation may be done either independently or in conjunction with mental health professionals or educators. In some ways, book discussions can provide a less threatening environment for discussion because comments can focus on characters or incidents in the materials and thus remain less personal. One librarian in South Carolina uses modern young adult novels to promote discussion between parents and their teenagers. Suicide, drugs, and premarital sex are some of the topics covered. When the young people involved are themselves displaying or likely to display risky behavior, a mental health professional should be an integral part of the discussion team.

Some children or young adults, and some topics, are more sensitive or delicate than others. In these cases, the librarian's background enables him or her to be a productive, contributing member of a team working to help these young people.

Booktalks

A *booktalk* is a formal speech about books and other materials. Often centered on a theme, the intent of a booktalk is to entice listeners to read the book, view the video, or listen to the recording. The librarian or media specialist uses selection and evaluation skills to identify titles suitable for the planned presentation. Then he or she deliberately talks about the item in such a way and in just enough detail to "hook" the listeners. The ending is rarely told and the audience is often left hanging at the most exciting part of the story. Library professionals often know from personal experience how successful booktalks can be in generating reader interest. As Chelton stated, "Skill in booktalking remains one of the most valuable promotional devices Young Adult librarians can have at hand" (Chelton 1980, 503).

Potential topics for booktalking are limitless. Examples pertinent to bibliotherapy may range from making friends to sibling rivalry to peer pressure to suicide to grief. The youth librarian can build on the selected theme to identify specific titles (fiction or nonfiction) in a variety of formats: print, video, or audio. Then he or she decides on a presentation order, identifies points to share from each title, prepares transitional statements between titles, and gets ready to give the booktalk. This booktalk can serve as an introduction to the topic or be a concluding activity. In either case, it is a good way to introduce children or young adults to a variety of pertinent titles.

Youth librarians regularly present booktalks as part of their work with children and young adults. Brief, informal booktalks are commonly part of reader's advisory. Moreover, public librarians and school library media specialists frequently booktalk titles in their own libraries or go to visit school classrooms. In 1980, Joni Bodart wrote the first of a series of books with suggestions on technique, which also includes sample booktalks (Bodart 1980).

This type of oral, personal presentation can work well as part of bibliotherapy sessions with groups of young people. First, the professional librarians and mental health personnel identify the topic. Next, the librarian or media specialist selects materials and prepares and presents the booktalk. Then both library and mental health professionals work with young people to discuss the material and explore any related issues. This technique could also be integrated into a school district's affective education program or around themes that were introduced in a therapeutic group led by a counselor, psychologist, or social worker.

CONCLUSION

In the public library or school library media center collection are many materials that can be used successfully with young people in bibliotherapy sessions. Furthermore, the library professionals who work there are willing and even eager to help children, young adults, and adults identify, locate, use, and enjoy the materials available. Therefore, the trained librarian's or library media specialist's skills may be adapted to and effectively support the practice of bibliotherapy.

REFERENCES

American Association of School Librarians and Association for Educational Communications and Technology. 1988. *Information Power: Guidelines for School Library Media Programs.* Chicago: American Library Association; Washington, DC: Association for Educational Communications and Technology, p. 20.

Barron, Pamela, and Jennifer Q. Burely. 1984. *Jump over the Moon: Study Guide.* New York: Holt, Rinehart, & Winston, pp. 62–63.

Benne, Mae. 1991. *Principles of Children's Services in Public Libraries.* Chicago: American Library Association, p. 2.

Billings, Harold. 1995. "The Tomorrow Librarian." *Wilson Library Bulletin* (January): 34–37.

Bodart, Joni. 1980. *Booktalk! Booktalking and School Visiting for Young Adult Audiences.* New York: H. W. Wilson.

Chelton, Mary K. 1980. "Booktalking: You Can Do It." In *Young Adult Literature: Background and Criticism,* comp. Millicent Lenz and Ramona M. Mahood. Chicago: American Library Association, p. 503.

Connor, Jane Gardner. 1985. *Children's Services Handbook.* Columbia: South Carolina State Library, pp. 2–44.

Fasick, Adele M. 1991. *Managing Children's Services in the Public Library.* Englewood, CO: Libraries Unlimited, p. 8.

Fitzgibbons, Shirley A. 1986. "Reference and Information Services for Children and Young Adults: Definition, Services, and Issues." In *Reference and Information Services: A Reader for Today,* comp. Bill Katz. Metuchen, NJ: Scarecrow Press.

Genco, Barbara A., Eleanor K. MacDonald, and Betsy Hearne. 1991. "Juggling Popularity and Quality." *School Library Journal* 37(3): 115–19.

Harrington, Janice N. 1985. "Reference Service in the Children's Department: A Case Study." *Public Library Quarterly* 6(3): 65–75.

Heins, Ethel L. 1982. " 'Go and Catch a Falling Star': What Is a Good Children's Book?" *Theory into Practice* 21(4): 247–53.

Horning, Kathleen T. 1994. "How Can I Help You? The Joys and Challenges of Reference Work with Children." *Show-Me Libraries* (Spring/Summer): 9–19.

Jennerich, Elaine Zaremba, and Edward J. Jennerich. 1987. *The Reference Interview as a Creative Art.* Littleton, CO: Libraries Unlimited.

Karl, Jean. 1982. "An Editor's View: Recognizing the Best." *Theory into Practice* 21(4): 254–61.

Lukens, Rebecca J. 1995. A *Critical Handbook of Children's Literature*, 5th ed. New York: HarperCollins.

Moores, Alan, and Rhea Rubin. 1984. *Let's Talk About It: A Planner's Manual.* Chicago: American Library Association.

Paterson, Katherine. 1977. *Bridge to Terabithia.* New York: Crowell.

Radford, Marie L. 1989. "Interpersonal Communication Theory in the Library Context: A Review of Current Perspectives." In *Library and Information Science Annual,* 5th ed., ed. Bohdan S. Wynar. Englewood, CO: Libraries Unlimited, pp. 3–10.

Rylant, Cynthia. 1992. *Missing May.* New York: Orchard Books.

Sexton, Kathryn. 1977. "The Reference Interview and the Young Adult." In *The Librarian and Reference Service,* selected by Arthur Ray Rowland. Hamden, CT: Shoe String Press, pp. 174–78.

U.S. Department of Education, Office of Educational Research and Improvement. 1988. *Services and Resources for Young Adults in Public Libraries.* National Center for Education Statistics: Survey Report 8.

———. 1990. *Services and Resources for Children in Public Libraries, 1988–89.* National Center for Education Statistics: Survey Reports 5.

Washington Library Association, Children's and Young Adult Services. 1989. *Advocating Access: Developing Community Library Services to Children and Young Adults in Washington State,* p. 14.

Zolotow, Charlotte. 1982. "Something That Makes Childhood Less Lonely." *Theory into Practice* 21(4): 263–64.

5 Skills of the Mental Health Professional

Communities provide mental health services to children and youth through a dizzying array of agencies, clinics, and professions. The therapist who sits across from a child may be trained as a psychologist, social worker, counselor or counseling psychologist, psychiatric nurse, or a psychiatrist. Any of these professions may be employed in schools, in which case they would typically be titled school psychologist, school counselor, school nurse, or school social worker. Additionally, some special education teachers specialize in instruction of children with emotional and behavioral disabilities. Each profession has a different historical origin and each professional will have somewhat different training experiences. Still, many mental health specialists believe that the services they provide are more alike than they are different (Drum 1987; Fox, Kovacs, and Graham 1985). We refer to these professionals jointly as *child therapists*.

Despite their diverse titles, child therapists share some common and essential skills. They are knowledgeable about the social and emotional development of both typical children and children with emotional disturbances. They know the home and community conditions that worsen children's mental health problems and often can identify children in the early stages of distress, before mental disorders become severe. When treatment is necessary, child therapists

49

are skilled at sorting through the various concerns about a child to clarify the essential problem; at helping children reflect upon and change their attitudes, grow in insight, or acquire new understandings; and at helping children use that insight to make real changes in their behavior. Because they also know the kinds of adult support that children and youth need for healthy social and emotional development, they can help parents, educators, and other adults be more supportive of children's mental health. When children or adolescents are struggling with serious mental health problems, child therapists recognize the signs and know which kinds of therapy are most likely to help a child cope or even recover. Because they understand and can negotiate the mental health service system, child therapists know who to contact and what to do to secure the therapeutic services that children or adolescents need.

It is child therapists, then, who can link a program of bibliotherapy into a school or community mental health system. Their participation can ensure that children or adolescents with serious emotional problems are identified early and provided with a program of services that will be effective for them. With youth whose distress is less marked, they can monitor the progress of bibliotherapy to ensure that it assuages rather than adds to their distress. They can act as a resource to children whose responses to literature are unusually intense, unanticipated, and painful. Child therapists can ensure that children act upon the personal insight and interpersonal understanding they gain through bibliotherapy and can monitor children's progress over time to ensure that this impact is lasting and meaningful. When included from the inception of a program's planning, they can enhance the program's fit with the mental health needs of a particular community's children. Alternatively, the contributions of media specialists can allow the child therapist to infuse high-quality literature and film into existing programs of therapeutic services, enhancing the services' believability and impact.

WHO ARE THE MENTAL HEALTH PROFESSIONALS?

Six types of mental health professionals are described here: psychologists, counselors or counseling psychologists, social workers, teachers of students with emotional disabilities, school or psychiatric nurses, and psychiatrists. Credentials and licensing for each are regulated separately by the states. Each profession is subject to somewhat different standards of training, is licensed with a different credential, and is governed by a different regulatory board. A community may also include a number of unlicensed persons who work to support the mental health of children and adolescents. Because it is difficult to differentiate between what is therapy and what is simple care and nurturing, it has been impossible to restrict the practices of lay professionals who do not meet the certification standards for the traditional mental health professions. Instead, most states regulate the mental health titles—that is, who can call themselves psychologists or social workers— rather than restricting the practices of counseling and therapy.

Psychologists

The title *licensed psychologist* is usually restricted to those who have completed a doctoral degree and a year of clinical internship in one of the four specialty areas of applied psychology: school psychology, clinical psychology, counseling psychology, or industrial/organizational psychology (Fox, Kovacs, and Graham 1985). Only specialists in the first three areas are likely to be working with children and adolescents. Professional training in applied psychology typically includes the study of social and biological bases of behavior, methods of psychological research, and psychological assessment and interventions for clients. Certain mental health workers may, instead, have earned master's degrees in the practice of psychology, and their work typically is supervised by a licensed psychologist. Psychology was a discipline of research and scholarship before it was an applied profession; traditionally, therefore, psychologists' practice differed from that of other mental health professionals in its emphasis on research-based evaluation of mental abilities and on empirically validated approaches to therapy. Now, research is integral to all of the mental health professions.

School Counselors and School Psychologists

Some school counselors and school psychologists are licensed psychologists, but others are certified or licensed by a state's educational agency to practice within the schools, and in this case may not have completed a doctorate. School counselors' training is most often forty-eight graduate semester hours that focus on development and integration of guidance programs into the school curriculum: counseling skills for individuals, groups, and families; career and vocational guidance; and counseling strategies for specific problems such as substance abuse, eating disorders, and attention deficit/hyperactivity disorder (Council for the Accreditation of Counseling and Related Educational Programs 1994). School psychologists complete a minimum of sixty graduate semester hours of training, including instruction in: psychotherapeutic interventions for individuals, groups, and classrooms; application of behavioral principles to individual, class, and systems management; research in development, learning theories, and social and biological bases of behavior; assessment methods; and consultation (National Association of School Psychologists 1994). Located in schools, both school counselors and school psychologists are likely to focus on the educational, as well as the social and emotional, needs of children and adolescents.

Licensed Professional Counselors

Many states also license professional counselors. Criteria for licensure vary widely from state to state, but generally require forty-eight graduate semester hours of coursework, including training in counseling theories and techniques, group counseling, and multicultural counseling. Subsequently, most states require that counselors pass the National Board Counseling Examination and complete two years of full-time practice under supervision, typically in a community mental health center or medical facility. Traditionally, services of licensed professional counselors focus on enhancing personal adjustment and supporting clients in their self-improvement efforts. The specific strategies used tend to be pragmatic and address day-to-day problems of clients.

Social Workers

Most social workers have completed a two-year master's degree program that includes coursework in community and family contributions, personal adjustment, and supervised fieldwork in a broad range of community services. Then, to practice privately in a community and earn a license as a clinical social worker, most social workers are required by the state to complete an additional two years of supervised clinical experience and pass an examination. Historically, social workers worked within communities to help families meet their needs for shelter, food, and clothing, in addition to providing emotional and social support. Contemporary roles for social workers incorporate considerable experience in therapeutic services for children and youth, remediating familial dysfunctions, and intervening in cases of family violence or poverty. Because they frequently work in medical settings, social workers are often trained in psychiatric diagnosis procedures.

Teachers of Students with Emotional Disabilities

Although teachers of students with emotional disabilities may be trained at the bachelor's level, most have earned a master's degree in special education. Their training provides them with special expertise in teaching children and adolescents with emotional or behavioral disorders, including strategies for individualizing instruction for students' special learning needs, managing students' volatile behavior and emotionality during instruction, providing extraordinary social and emotional support to students, utilizing systematic behavior management strategies, and providing skilled instruction in social and emotional competencies. As teachers, they are licensed or certified through a state's education agency and work primarily in schools or residential treatment facilities for youth.

Psychiatrists and Psychiatric Nurses

Psychiatrists are physicians who have completed a three-year residency in psychiatry following their medical training. Psychiatrists receive extensive training in psychiatric diagnosis as well as therapy services, and are the only mental health professionals authorized to prescribe medication for mental disorders. Psychiatric nurses are registered nurses who often have a master's degree in mental health. In medical settings, psychiatric nurses may provide the majority of the direct care to clients. Additionally, in some cases *school nurses* are employed by school districts to provide health services. Although primarily trained in physical health, nurses often become important members of school mental health teams because of their expertise in such issues as teen pregnancy, sexuality, and substance abuse.

HOW MENTAL HEALTH SERVICES ARE PROVIDED TO CHILDREN AND ADOLESCENTS

Children are usually brought to the attention of a child therapist by a teacher, parent, or other adult caretaker, although by adolescence some youths will refer themselves to therapists, seeking help with their distress. In most cases, the referrals are prompted by the youth's misbehavior. Achenbach (1991) reports that over half of the referrals to child guidance centers were due to children's noncompliant and disruptive behavior. Child therapists begin by gathering information about the child's social and emotional difficulties. Using their knowledge of the signs of social and emotional distress, they interview parents, collect reports and ratings about the child's behavior, and interview and observe the child directly. Often, their careful examination will show that the caretaker's real concern was somewhat different than was originally stated, or that the youth is experiencing multiple problems that may aggravate each other. Once the information is collected, child therapists will compare it to typical patterns of social and emotional development to decide whether the child is experiencing one of the many normal problems that all children struggle with, or whether the difficulties are unusually severe or long-lasting and so require special intervention.

Because children's problems are not always caused by their own pathology, a child therapist will also collect information about the adults who are responsible for the children's care and the home, school, or community situations in which they live. Events that are all-too-typical in today's families, including divorce, remarriage, a parent's illness, or the death of a grandparent, can be traumatic for children and can diminish the quality of care that a parent is able to provide (Doll 1996b). Communities, too, can disrupt a child's socioemotional equilibrium if they are excessively violent, overcrowded, or impose unrealistic and harsh expectations for child behavior. The social climate created by children's peers can contribute to their unhappiness and loneliness, when they are not well accepted or chosen as friends, or can contribute to their resilience by providing them with a source of support, companionship, and understanding (Doll 1996a). Even if the problem appears to originate with the child, these contexts can contribute to or protect a child from life stresses. A broad understanding of the child that includes these factors can provide child therapists with sources of support and assistance that they can integrate into their intervention plan.

Deciding when therapy is necessary is also important. A delicate balance exists between the benefits of providing a child with an additional source of assistance and the disruption caused by marking the child as different or in need of help. Therapists often solve this dilemma by working through parents or teachers instead. In the attempt to remediate a child's difficulties, a therapist might help caretakers plan new ways to respond to misbehavior or of encouraging a child to be more active or outgoing. The therapist might teach caretakers new skills—ways of listening more carefully to what a child says, ways of running a family meeting to talk about problems and make decisions, or ways of controlling the child during a temper tantrum. In other cases, the therapist provides new knowledge about children and their development to enhance caretakers' ability to counsel a child. For example, one therapy group teaches parents about children's friendships and suggests ways that adults can assist children who are without friends (Doll 1996a). When the therapist believes that poor quality of care is contributing to the child's problems, he or she might also recommend a program of ongoing consultation with caretakers instead of direct services to the child.

If therapists decide to work directly with the child, they might choose from a variety of different techniques, each defended by different theoretical perspectives. Behavioral therapists describe children's social and emotional adjustment in terms of the behaviors that children perform and the ways that parents and others in the child's social world prompt these behaviors and respond to them (Mash and Barkley 1989). To intervene, behavioral therapists are likely to suggest that the consequences of children's behavior be altered in carefully planned ways to shape alternative and more adaptive behaviors on the part of the child. For example, a behavioral therapist might suggest that a parent ignore a child's interruptions during parental phone conversations in order to discourage that behavior in the future. Conversely, a behavioral therapist might help a teacher establish a program of rewarding a child's work completion with extra recess time. At other times, a behavioral therapist might work directly to teach a child self-management skills, including self-observation, self-recording of behavior changes, and self-rewarding of positive behaviors.

Gestalt therapists believe that children's social and emotional adjustment emerges out of their past experiences—experiences that have shaped their beliefs about why people react to them in certain ways and what they can do to change those reactions. Gestalt therapists are likely to guide children through a set of carefully planned activities that allow them to reexperience people in new ways and to alter their expectations of others, and thus change the way they enter into or initiate experiences (Oaklander 1978). For example, a gestalt therapist might help children visualize themselves as strong and effective leaders as a way of empowering them to confront teasing from their peers.

Humanistic therapists believe that children's natural inclination to be content and well adjusted is disrupted when adults threaten disapproval or even dislike of them. Humanistic therapists will work to create an experience in which the child feels accepted and valued, to enhance the child's adjustment. Humanistic therapists actively listen to children's descriptions of themselves and their beliefs, subtly leading them to discover their strengths and competencies. Moreover, a humanistic therapist would recommend that parents actively listen to and authentically praise their children, so that the young people will feel accepted and free to explore their individuality.

Cognitive therapists believe that children's ways of acting originate in their cognitive understanding of themselves and of others. The cognitive therapist will work to help children acquire knowledge and garner new understanding of themselves and what they are capable of (Hughes 1988; Kendall and Braswell 1985). Cognitive therapists are likely to assist children in understanding the perspective of the other children with whom they argue, as one strategy to sensitize them to the need to adjust their behavior to that of others. Alternatively, cognitive therapists might teach children to use self-talk to guide their actions or decision making. One prominent cognitive strategy is to teach children systematic problem-solving steps to use when making a decision: identifying and describing the problem, listing several alternative actions that they might take, explaining the possible consequences of each choice, choosing one alternative and trying it out, and evaluating the plan to decide whether it was successful.

Psychoeducational interventions are likely to be used in schools or residential treatment programs; these are instructional programs that teach children specific knowledge or psychosocial skills calculated to reduce their problems (Elias and Tobias 1996, Goldstein 1988). For example, children might be taught specific steps for negotiating a compromise with another child and given an opportunity to practice those steps in role-plays or simulations. Or children might be taught systematic relaxation techniques and given an explanation of when and how to use them. Other psychoeducational programs have been developed to teach children to stop and think rather than acting impulsively, to mediate conflicts between other children, to stop bullying in their classrooms, to reduce the stress in their lives, and to manage anger effectively.

Many child therapists endorse an eclectic combination of different theories, and so will combine alternative intervention strategies into a menu or combination of techniques. Although research often shows that one form of therapy is more effective than another for particular psychological disorders, there is good evidence demonstrating that different child therapies are equally effective.

Whatever the therapeutic model, all effective child therapists work carefully to ensure that children act upon the insight and enhanced understanding they gain from therapy. In most cases, it is important for therapists to verify that the child's actual behavior improves in the everyday settings where it was previously problematic. Using various monitoring techniques and different indices of change, they check and recheck to see that the advances children make persist and even deepen. Then they check back to ensure that these changes do not disappear after the therapy has ended. Propelling children into making changes, and ensuring that these changes become solidified as part of the child's habitual ways of being, are the hallmark of effective therapy.

LINKING BIBLIOTHERAPY WITH THERAPEUTIC INTERVENTIONS

The personal insight, emotional catharsis, and interpersonal understanding that emerge from the act of reading can be integrated into ongoing programs of child therapy in several different ways. First, the personal insight that readers achieve can be captured and become the basis for self-understanding and subsequent self-change. A deeper self-understanding can make children more receptive to a therapist's suggestions about the reasons for their problems, the ways in which they might themselves contribute to their difficulties, and the steps they might take to correct the problems. Child therapists can then follow this insight with systematic strategies to implement, monitor, and fine-tune the plans that children have made.

The different characters portrayed in fictional work can act as models for the social skills that a child needs to acquire. Characters who act out the systematic problem-solving steps, respond in assertive ways to bullies, or take the risky step of inviting another child to play can be copied by readers who find themselves in similar situations. The conversations between fictional characters, or the effective comebacks characters use in difficult social situations, can be used as conversational scripts for a child to follow. Child therapists can use these models as both good and bad examples of the social skills they are attempting to teach. Moreover, the scenarios that are portrayed in children's literature can serve as scenes for role-playing activities between child therapists and children. Because they are rich in descriptions of the context of a situation, the role-playing scenarios derived from literature will be more effective and more realistic than those found in most psychoeducational curricula.

One recurring dilemma faced by child therapists is that children's most intense and difficult emotions often occur outside the therapy room, and so cannot be addressed directly. Literature and film, with their ability to elicit authentic and actual feelings from the reader or viewer, hold the potential for bringing this emotional experience back into the treatment. Then the child therapist can use this opportunity to guide the child through accurate interpretations of the feeling and its cause, and to develop effective strategies for expressing and controlling the emotion in ways that do not get the child into trouble. Moreover, the cathartic relief that emerges when a person is able to experience intense emotion in very safe circumstances can add to the child's relief.

Finally, children are often relieved to understand that they are not the only ones undergoing the feelings and facing the difficulties that they are facing. One of the authors will never forget the amazement and relief of one autistic sixth-grader when he realized that there were other children like him in the world—that he was not alone. Recognizing the commonalities of their experiences provides children with an opportunity to view themselves from another perspective—that of a group with common characteristics, and frees them from the pervasive self-blame that often blocks their movement into healthier ways of being.

Each of these factors also holds some risk. Children may not identify with the competent and healthy characters of a fictional work, and so may find themselves modeling the behaviors and attitudes of characters who are unsuccessful and unhealthy. The emotional impact of a novel could exaggerate and intensify children's emotional experiences, especially when they have not directly addressed the issues underlying their feelings. The distorted insights that children gain about others or themselves could be inaccurate or even harmful. By working in partnerships of media specialists and child therapists, however, these risks can be addressed quickly and effectively.

REFERENCES

Achenbach, T. M. 1991. *Manual for the Children Behavior Checklist/4–18*. Burlington: University of Vermont.

Council for the Accreditation of Counseling and Related Educational Programs. 1994. *CACREP Accreditation Standards and Procedures Manual*. Alexandria, VA: Author.

Doll, B. 1996a. "Children Without Friends: Implications for Practice and Policy." *School Psychology Review* 25: 165–83.

———. 1996b. "Prevalence of Psychiatric Disorders in Children and Youth: An Agenda for Advocacy by School Psychology." *School Psychology Quarterly* 11: 1–27.

Drum, D. J. 1987. "Do We Have a Multiple Personality?" *Counseling Psychologist* 15: 337–40.

Elias, Maurice J., and Steven E. Tobias. 1996. *Social Problem Solving: Interventions in the Schools*. New York: Guilford Press.

Fox, R. E., A. L. Kovacs, and S. R. Graham. 1985. "Proposals for a Revolution in the Preparation and Regulation of Professional Psychologists." *American Psychologist* 40: 1042–50.

Goldstein, A. P. 1988. *The Prepare Curriculum*. Champaign, IL: Research Press.

Hughes, J. N. 1988. *Cognitive Behavior Therapy with Children in Schools*. New York: Pergamon Press.

Kendall, P. C., and L. Braswell. 1985. *Cognitive-Behavioral Therapy for Impulsive Children*. New York: Guilford Press.

Mash, E. J., and R. A. Barkley. 1989. *Treatment of Childhood Disorders*. New York: Guilford Press.

National Association of School Psychologists. 1994. *The Standards for Training and Field Placement Programs in School Psychology*. Washington, DC: Author.

Oaklander, V. 1978. *Windows to Our Children*. Moab, UT: Real People Press.

6 Cautions for Bibliotherapy Leaders

Marsha Wiggins Frame and Beth Doll

The idea of literature as a therapeutic instrument can be compelling, possibly because those who choose to engage others in bibliotherapy have found that books provide insight and meaning for their own lives. However, precisely because of its usefulness in helping young people wrestle with their dilemmas, some words of caution and direction must be offered to librarians and media specialists who may be conducting their programs without the immediate participation of a mental health professional. This chapter offers some general cautions regarding bibliotherapy and then describes a continuum of emotional and behavioral reactions that professionals may encounter when working with children and adolescents. It also indicates what kinds of action leaders of developmental bibliotherapy should take in response to these reactions.

CAUTIONS IN SELECTING MATERIALS

It is essential to remember that everyone, no matter how young, brings a personal life history to a story. Readers use their own experiences and their ways of making sense out of those experiences as the backdrop for a bibliotherapist's tales. Then, whenever adults share a book with a young person, they are entering into that child's world, complete with the fear, worry, sadness, joy, or excitement that lies beneath the surface. Good stories have the power to evoke intense emotional responses from listeners in part because they involve these potent and very personal experiences from the past. Bibliotherapy leaders need to be alert to these emotional responses of the audience and to recognize when the responses are so intense or painful as to overpower the listener (Halliday 1991). Also, to be helpful, bibliotherapy leaders need to introduce a variety of ways for their hearers to interpret the stories, thus moving them into new understandings of their own lives.

Professionals must also attend to the solutions provided for the problems their books address. Some popular stories offer simplistic or "band-aid" solutions that do little to assist children or adolescents in dealing with complex, real-life problems (Chatton 1988). When these simplified solutions are ultimately unsuccessful, young readers can become discouraged and give up prematurely in their attempts to deal with important personal problems. Conversely, other books present characters who must struggle with an array of problems. These multifaceted challenges may enhance the plot, but they may also be emotionally overwhelming to hearers (Chatton 1988). Such books can convey the message that problems like these are too difficult to resolve successfully. The skilled group leader can use discussion time to correct for both of these literary weaknesses, by questioning how realistic it is to expect such simple solutions to work, or by pointing out ways in which the story either oversimplified real-world dilemmas or magnified them.

Another important challenge facing professionals is that of managing values—those implicit in the books they use or their own. Some books that are frequently used for therapeutic purposes embody humanistic values, but others are laden with imagery or outcomes that are violent, racist, sexist, ageist, or otherwise insensitive to the values held by young listeners and adult professionals. Other times, in an effort to be helpful, leaders' interpretations of stories may unnecessarily impose their own dearly held values on young listeners. For example, if a book's story line includes a child or adolescent whose parents are separated or divorced, the casual comments of a leader who believes that divorce is wrong could inadvertently increase the young person's distress or guilt. Thus, it is important that bibliotherapy leaders become sensitive to the values espoused in the books recommended for use in bibliotherapy. It is also necessary for professionals to monitor their own values vis-à-vis the literature they select to share with children and young adults. Self-scrutiny is important because it prevents professionals from using literature as a personal forum, at the expense of assisting their listeners to formulate their own ideas and draw their own conclusions from the stories.

COMMON SIGNS OF DISTRESS

Whether librarians and media specialists or mental health personnel, leaders of bibliotherapy will encounter a variety of behaviors and emotional responses from children and young adults when they discuss and share thought-provoking literature with those children. Several major themes emerge: restlessness, behaving like younger children, fearfulness, withdrawal, complaints of illness, emotional outbursts, and talk of suicide. All of these expressions fall on a continuum from ordinary to severe. These behaviors and emotional responses are described here, along with recommendations for the bibliotherapist's course of action.

Restlessness

Restlessness is one of the most common signs of distress that bibliotherapy leaders may notice among the children and adolescents in their audience. Some fidgeting and poking of others are normal and should be expected when children are assembled in large groups. As a convenient rule of thumb, children can easily attend to a story for approximately five minutes for every year of age over three (Barkley 1990). For example, that means that one could expect six-year-olds to attend to a fifteen-minute story, especially if they are accustomed to sitting and listening. When children cannot listen quietly for a reasonable amount of time, adults should first examine whether the location or timing of the discussion is contributing to their restlessness. For example, children will struggle more to pay attention when rooms are too hot, when they are hungry, or immediately before a major holiday. Changing the room or providing a snack may be all that is needed to improve the attention of children and adolescents.

In some cases, children's restlessness and fidgety behaviors are extreme—they are in constant motion. There may be a driven quality to their movement and their antics interrupt the group seemingly without control. Children and adolescents who struggle with attention deficit disorders can show this pattern of overactivity, especially as the discussion sessions lengthen and other children linger over topics (Barkley 1990). When attention deficits have not been diagnosed, restlessness this pronounced may signal a less visible emotional turmoil that could be entirely unrelated to the bibliotherapy program. However, if the overactivity waxes and wanes depending on the topic of the story being discussed or the issues that a story line raises, the book itself may be feeding the turmoil. Adults' first inclination when working with children this disruptive is to become irritated and to harshly reprimand the child. Indeed, such children are lectured so frequently and severely about their misbehaviors that they often carry emotional scars that feed their discouragement. Evidence has shown that discipline is more likely to be effective when the consequences of misbehavior are mild but very consistently applied (Forehand and McMahon 1981). Moreover, when working with children who exhibit signs of more serious distress and cannot attend to the reading or discussion of selected literature, librarians and media specialists should consult with both mental health professionals and parents early and often, to alert them to the behaviors and to develop effective responses to the behaviors.

Between normal restlessness on one end of the continuum and the endless movement of seriously anxious children are behaviors that indicate moderate distress. For example, some children or adolescents may be impulsive, blurting out ideas or answers out of turn or engaging in pesky, irritating interactions with children sitting nearby. Such occasional fidgeting is no cause for alarm, and could serve important purposes for the child—securing much-needed attention from the leader or their peers. They may also be acting disruptively to distract themselves or to escape from a particularly poignant scene of a book. When struggling with such mild disruption and distractions, bibliotherapy leaders might first ask the child to decide how the problem should be handled. Alternatively, parents, teachers, or mental health professionals who are familiar with the child might know how this behavior has been handled successfully in other settings.

In a few, very rare cases, some of the restlessness that children and adolescents demonstrate will be part of a set of elaborate rituals they feel compelled to act out (Flament et al. 1988). For example, the rituals might govern how they enter or leave a room or how the furniture has to be placed. Other children may incessantly wash their hands or other objects whenever they come in contact with the floor, another person, or an object. They check to be sure clothing and belongings are intact, count objects or words, or recite ritualistic phrases. Although these kinds of behaviors typically do not originate in the books and videos to which children are exposed, such actions indicate serious distress and should prompt an immediate referral to mental health specialists. At the same time, such rituals are generally not good reason to exclude children from a bibliotherapy program that is otherwise enjoyable to them, especially if the other participants in the group can accept the rituals' strangeness without ostracizing the child.

Behaving Like Much Younger Children

It is common for children, and less common for adolescents, to revert to behaviors typical of younger children when they are distressed. Bibliotherapy leaders might observe minor regressive behaviors such as thumbsucking, cuddling, or fearfulness, especially during frightening moments in a story's plot. When these relapses are fleeting and mild, they have served their purpose in providing temporary comfort to the child and should not be of concern. Instead, the leader can make a mental note of a child's reactions and continue to watch for the behavior in subsequent sessions. However, if older children or adolescents exhibit highly regressive behaviors more than five years distant from their actual age (especially when wetting or soiling is evident in children older than seven years), both parents and mental health professionals should be alerted immediately.

Fearfulness

All children go through phases of being afraid of things—of being in the dark, monsters, or being abandoned by their caretakers (Morris and Kratochwill 1983). Indeed, some children are temperamentally more fearful than their peers and will be easily distressed by plot lines that their friends find amusing. Though some will describe their fears directly and easily, others will mask them by laughing uncontrollably or becoming very silent. Fears become concerning when their intensity is out of proportion to the actual danger the child is in, and when they prevent children from going places or doing things that they would otherwise enjoy. Thus, professionals would be wise to alert parents when children demonstrate uncontrollable distress in which they cannot be comforted and that prevents them from exploring a book or plot that most children find enjoyable.

Complaints of Illness

Should discussions, videos, or books become too upsetting, some children will begin to complain of minor illnesses or have recurring somatic complaints such as headaches or stomachaches. Often these physical complaints occur during emotionally laden moments in a book, only to recede once the mood lightens or the critical issue resolves. Many times, these symptoms serve the purpose of excusing the child from the group (a hidden form of withdrawal) or securing additional comfort from the group's leader. In this situation, the physical complaints may become more pronounced or more frequent during tense moments in a story's plot. When the symptoms are frequent or persist over time, the bibliotherapist might confer with parents and teachers to determine if these symptoms are also evident in other settings.

Emotional Outbursts

One of the meaningful characteristics of good literature is its power to move us to tears. Emotional expressions like tears are normal reactions to moving moments of novels. In lieu of tears, books may elicit young persons' worries or deep sadness, or prompt them to reexperience life events of which the book characters have reminded them. At the same time, books can elicit unexpected joy and contentment or other rewarding emotional moments. Bibliotherapy leaders expect books to be emotionally expansive for their readers and so presume that these cathartic occurrences will happen. The emotionality of literature can be problematic for children or adolescents who are so focused on negative thoughts that they become morose and even hostile. They may weep uncontrollably, isolate themselves from the group, or even wildly dominate a discussion. If a child or adolescent becomes emotionally distraught to the point of not being able to compose himself or herself, and does not respond to comforting by adults or peers, librarians and media specialists should encourage parents to consult with a mental health professional immediately.

Talk of Suicide

When a book's themes are morose or discouraging, or if they trigger disheartening memories from children's pasts, comments about suicide may emerge during a discussion group. Participants may disclose that they have thought about killing themselves, or may make vague statements such as, "Nobody cares about me. I might as well end it all." They may even mention that they have known someone who completed suicide. Younger children may express a desire to be reunited with a loved one who has died. Given how common such suicidal ideations are among adolescents (see chapter 3), it is quite likely that others in the discussion group have thought about suicide without revealing it out loud. The wisest course of action is not to pursue the suicidal comments within the whole group, but to alert the parents immediately about their child's suicidal remarks. If the children's comments reveal that they have made detailed and realistic plans for suicide, or that they have taken steps to complete the plans, librarians and media specialists should consult immediately with mental health professionals to determine whether the child should be detained while parents are informed of the risk.

Discouragement

Between the one who cries at a moving episode and the despondent or suicidal participant lies a child or adolescent who is moderately discouraged. These young people may appear to be tired or lethargic. They may express pessimism regarding the outcome of a book or their own circumstances. They may respond irritably when asked a question or when interacting with peers. One also may notice that such a child or adolescent is unable to concentrate and may momentarily "check out" of a segment of a book. Some vague thoughts about suicide may be expressed. However, this type of moderately distressed person will not exhibit a clear, detailed plan for suicide. The perceptive leader will want to monitor such a child or adolescent's behavior and consult with parents and mental health professionals regarding possible referral for mental health services.

OTHER SIGNS OF RISK

Concerns with weight. Preoccupation with food and weight is a hallmark of American culture. From an early age, girls in particular are focused on maintaining an ideal body image. It is not uncommon to hear elementary-school-age girls discussing the fat content of foods or expressing concern about weight gain. These fixations often emerge during book discussions when a book's characters are similarly preoccupied with eating or struggling with being overweight. It is important to notify parents immediately should the discussion reveal any dangerous purging, overexercise, or laxative use to restrict weight gain (described in chapter 3).

Inappropriate conduct. Another set of behaviors that can be of concern to professionals are those that include conflict and inappropriate conduct. It is typical to find children and/or adolescents engaging in mutual fighting and teasing and ignoring limits that are not clearly enforced. It would not be out of the ordinary to find some children rummaging through a desk or purse or taking all the books or toys off a shelf. Similarly, it is common to observe some children pushing and shoving each other and bandying about minor insults. Any bibliotherapist working with children or adolescents in groups should be prepared to manage this kind of misbehavior during the discussions. Nevertheless, one should be concerned about belligerent defiance of authority, angry outbursts (especially when limits are set), cruel bullying or assaultive behavior toward peers, or violation of laws. Children showing this pattern of cruelty may be beyond the scope of developmental bibliotherapy programs. It will be more difficult to decide how to respond to conduct problems that fall somewhere in between. These include children or adolescents who exhibit continual aggressive behavior, either verbal or physical. They may not back down when confronted by an adult and often have short tempers. If one observes this behavior, along with swearing or blaming others, it is important to consult with teachers and parents. If the behaviors escalate, bibliotherapy leaders might seek the assistance of mental health professionals to develop a more effective plan for managing group behavior.

When book discussions occur in groups, some children may become especially quiet or assume a daydream-like state while listening to a story. Perhaps the child is simply reflecting on what is being shared or is internally managing something mildly upsetting. At other times, children may be so emotionally distressed by a book's story that they simply "leave the room" at key moments. Temporary withdrawal is an effective coping strategy for children who are just learning to self-manage imposing emotional experiences. Unless the withdrawal persists or deepens, it should not be cause for alarm.

The quality of participants' peer relationships may also be significant to bibliotherapy leaders. These relationships may be a focus of considerable distress for some children and adolescents. Mild altercations and teasing are to be expected. Young people often express hurt feelings over being left out of a group or over sudden changes in friendships. These experiences are widespread and routine. However, bibliotherapists may observe that some children or adolescents are acutely and openly rejected by their peers (Doll 1996). They isolate themselves from peer interactions and may have only one or two acquaintances. They may be socially awkward, saying and doing things that offend or irritate their peers. This extreme peer rejection and isolation calls for parental involvement and for the bibliotherapy leader to seek aid from mental health professionals. Less distressed children and adolescents may engage in fighting and teasing behavior, but, beyond that, they may express excessive concerns about their friendship networks and about acceptance by peers. Although these children or adolescents may not need immediate mental health intervention, they are distressed by difficult peer relationships. Bibliotherapy leaders should consult with parents and teachers regarding this behavior pattern and offer these young people opportunities to interact with peers in a positive environment.

Family concerns may surface easily in the context of bibliotherapy, as many books and stories deal directly with family life and relationships. In a country where 50 percent of marriages fail, it is not unusual for children to express concern about the stability of their parents' marriages. They may verbalize these concerns or become anxious or distracted when the books or stories selected deal with issues of parental conflict or separation. The extreme behaviors mentioned previously, such as constant movement, leaving the room, making somatic complaints, and wetting or soiling, all suggest more distress than is typical for children dealing with a family transition. Again, bibliotherapy leaders would want to speak with parents if these danger signs are noted.

Finally, *child abuse* is another area of concern for those who work with children and adolescents in any capacity. Although it is not uncommon for parents to use corporal punishment, or for children to talk about being spanked, any punishment that results in marks, burns, bruises, or welts can be considered abusive and must be reported to child protective services if the group leader is a mandated reporter. (In most states, teachers, psychologists, counselors, and social workers are *mandated reporters* who are required to report any and all suspicions of child abuse [Fisher and Sorenson 1996]). Likewise, many preschool-age children are very interested in their own and others' genitalia and may engage in some exploratory sex play. If such an incident occurs during a bibliotherapy session, one can redirect the children's attention, pointing out that such behavior is inappropriate for reading time. If, however, children or adolescents disclose sexual activity with an adult or even another child five years (or more) their senior, this information, too, must be reported to child protective services.

CONCLUSION

Bibliotherapy provides an opportunity for those who love literature to use it as a vehicle for helping children and adolescents to deal with the problems of everyday living. Characters in books can normalize life's dilemmas and offer alternative solutions. Nevertheless, bibliotherapy also holds the potential for unleashing intense emotions and uncontrolled behaviors. It is critical that bibliotherapy leaders develop an ability to distinguish between behaviors that are common and expected and those that are indications of more serious distress. Bibliotherapy leaders need to sensitively address children and adolescents' minor concerns that may arise in the context of reading, and to seek assistance from mental health professionals when young people exhibit more severe behaviors. In this way, librarians and media specialists may work within the limits of their training and experience and the therapeutic enterprise may be fruitful and rewarding.

REFERENCES

Barkley, R. A. 1990. *Attention Deficit Hyperactivity Disorder: A Handbook for Diagnosis and Treatment.* New York: Guilford Press.

Chatton, Barbara. Spring 1988. "Apply with Caution: Bibliotherapy in the Library." *Journal of Youth Services in Libraries* 1(3): 334–38.

Doll, B. 1996. "Children Without Friends: Implications for Practice and Policy." *School Psychology Review* 25: 165–83.

Fisher, L., and G. P. Sorenson. 1996. *School Law for Counselors, Psychologists, and Social Workers,* 3rd ed. New York: Longman.

Flament, M. F., A. Whitaker, J. Rapoport, M. Davies, C. Zaremba, M. A. Berg, K. Kalikow, W. Sceery, and D. Schaffer. 1988. "Obsessive-compulsive Disorder in Adolescence: An Epidemiological Study." *Journal of the American Academy of Child and Adolescent Psychiatry* 27: 764–71.

Forehand, R., and R. J. McMahon. 1981. *Helping the Noncompliant Child: A Clinician's Guide to Parent Training.* New York: Guilford Press.

Halliday, G. 1991. "Psychological Self-Help Books—How Dangerous Are They?" *Psychology* 28(4): 678–80.

Morris, R. J., and T. R. Kratochwill. 1983. *Treating Children's Fears and Phobias.* New York: Pergamon Press.

7 Bibliographic Tools

The field of children's and young adult literature is rich in bibliographies and other guides to media. These tools provide excellent subject access to the world of books, audiovisual materials, and electronic media available for youth. Furthermore, many of these lists identify good, recommended titles. Librarians are aware of many of these sources and knowledgeable about their use, but mental health professionals may not be.

This chapter describes the type and variety of these bibliographies. Given the overwhelming number of these reference sources, no effort has been made to include every available bibliography in this chapter. Instead, the most recent editions of four standard selection tools were used to identify the twenty-two titles included here. These four tools were: *Elementary School Library Collection: A Guide to Books and Other Media* (Lee 1994); *Children's Catalog* (Yaakov 1991); *Junior High School Library Catalog* (Yaakov 1990); and *Senior High School Library Catalog* (Smith and Yaakov 1992). These books are updated on a two- to five-year cycle. Their purpose is to identify books and audiovisual or electronic materials currently in print that are recommended for inclusion in library collections for children and young adults. Titles are included for teachers, librarians, or other adults who help young people use library or media collections. Each reference title included in this chapter has been recommended in one or more of these four standard tools.

For each bibliography, a citation is given, followed by comments on the content, subjects, strengths, weaknesses, and limitations of the reference. Taken in their totality, the titles here demonstrate the range and diversity of bibliographic tools available. Many standard tools and classics in the field are here, and it is likely that readers will find specific sources they wish to consult. At the same time, readers are urged also to examine the four standard selection tools for additional sources that may meet the unique needs of their bibliotherapy program.

Each bibliography listed here has its own strengths and weaknesses. The organization of each differs, according to the method determined by its authors to be the most appropriate. Bibliotherapy leaders will use each in a slightly different way. These or similar tools are widely available in libraries. In situations where mental health professionals are working independently to provide a program of bibliotherapy, youth librarians can be consulted for additional guidance in locating and using such tools.

	Baskin, Barbara H., and Karen H. Harris. *More Notes from a Distant Drummer: A Guide to Juvenile Fiction Portraying the Disabled.* New York: R. R. Bowker, 1984.
Content Synopsis	This annotated guide to juvenile fiction that portrays characters with impairments was compiled to promote understanding of individuals so afflicted. The 348 titles, published between 1976 and 1981, are arranged alphabetically by author. Each title portrays at least one disabled character; disabilities cover visual, orthopedic, and auditory impairments.
Age Levels (as specified in the reference book)	5 to 18 years old
Indexes	Two indexes: title, subject
Content Parameters	• Only fiction titles written for juveniles • Excludes folklore, biographies, nonfiction, and novels from sectarian presses that expound a particular religious belief
Annotations	• Plot summaries focus on the role of the impairment and attitudes toward it • Analysis section evaluates the literary merit of the title and gives a critical assessment of the portrayal of the disabled characters or disability, including the tone and attitude conveyed toward the impairment
Strengths	• Includes titles from major genres, including contemporary, science fiction, fantasy, historical fiction, romance, and mystery • Detailed plot summaries

- Includes outline of Criteria for Selection of Intervention Strategy and discusses how literature can meet those criteria
- Chapter titled "Disabled in Literature" discusses trends and themes in the literature
- Reading-level designations not only describe appropriate ages and grades, but also include reading profiles indicating what a child or young adult is able to comprehend developmentally
- Distinguishes between impairment designations that play a central, critical role (all caps), and those that play a secondary role or have peripheral significance (lowercase)
- Addresses 10 disability designations: auditory impairment; cosmetic impairment; emotional dysfunction; intellectual impairment; learning disability; neurological impairment; orthopedic impairment; special health problems, such as cardiac disorders, rheumatism, and the like; speech impairment; and visual impairment
- Omits novels from sectarian presses that expound a particular religious belief

Weaknesses

- No list of recommended titles—reader must scan each analysis to determine if book is well written and gives an accurate portrayal
- Plot summaries are more extensive than the analysis section

---

Bernstein, Joanne E., and Masha Kabakow Rudman. *Books to Help Children Cope with Separation and Loss: An Annotated Bibliography.* Vol. 3. New York: R. R. Bowker, 1989.

Content Synopsis

This resource acts as a reference guide to help adults select fiction and nonfiction books for children on the themes of loss and separation. An introductory section provides background information on separation and loss for children and on bibliotherapy. This is followed by an annotated bibliography of 606 titles, which is divided into thematic categories, such as: Facing Separation; Different Kinds of Separation; Coping with Tragic Loss; and Adoption/Foster Care/Homelessness. A bibliography of selected references for adults is also included.

Age Levels (as specified in the reference book)	3 to 16 years
Indexes	Five indexes: author, title, subject, interest level, reading level
Content Parameters	• Books published from 1983 to 1988
Annotations	• Concise plot summaries and evaluation, with an emphasis on thematic issues • Notes the title's strengths and weaknesses, both as literature and as a "bibliotherapeutic medium"
Strengths	• Includes some titles published by small, specialized presses • Titles carefully selected for quality, lack of bias, and child appeal • Essays on separation and loss and on bibliotherapy • Indexes offer access by interest level and reading level
Weaknesses	• Primarily limited to realistic fiction

	Campbell, Patty. *Sex Guides: Books and Films About Sexuality for Young Adults.* New York: Garland Publications, 1986.
Content Synopsis	This source is designed to serve as a guide to sex manuals and materials that can be used to educate young adults about sex and sexuality. It traces the history of sex guides for adolescents up through the 1970s and discusses modern materials, including young adult fiction, religious sex prevention guides, sex guide spin-offs, audiovisual materials, and materials designed for parents, teachers, and librarians. A bibliography of recommended nonfiction and fiction titles for the junior high school library, the senior high school library, and the public library young adult sections is included. The author is a free-lance writer, critic, and general editor of Twayne's Young Adult Author series.
Age Levels (as specified in the reference book)	Young adults, age 11 to 18 years
Indexes	One index: author/title/subject
Content Parameters	• Books may be outdated, as titles were published from the late 1970s to mid-1980s

Annotations	• Evaluative and descriptive comments embedded in chapter discussions
	• Covers both recommended and not recommended titles
Strengths	• Emphasis on titles appropriate for library collections
	• Chapter on young adult fiction as sex education
	• Covers issues such as pregnancy, STDs, and homosexuality
	• Includes audiovisual materials
	• Includes an evaluation checklist for sex education materials
Weaknesses	• Amount of content information about each title varies
	• Recommended titles listed in appendix; must consult index for locations of annotations in previous chapters
	• Does not include religious guides from non-Western religions (limited to Christian and Jewish materials)

Charles, Sharon Ashenbrenner, and Sari Feldman. *Drugs: A Multimedia Sourcebook for Children and Young Adults.* New York: Neal Schuman, 1980.

Content Synopsis	As an evaluative resource of print and audiovisual materials for educating young people about drugs, this source aims to identify materials that are *not* judgmental, inaccurate, or insensitive. Fiction, nonfiction, and personal narrative titles are covered, as well as 16mm films and videos, audiocassettes and discs, filmstrips, sound/slide sets, and transparencies and slides. The following drugs are examined: marijuana, inhalants, PCP (phencyclidine), amphetamines, barbiturates, cocaine, alcohol, hallucinogens, and opium and its derivatives.
Age Levels (as specified in the reference book)	Grades 6 to 12
Indexes	Three indexes: author, title, subject
Content Parameters	• Materials published during the late 1960s through the 1970s

Annotations	• Content summaries and critical/evaluative comments
	• Where appropriate, reading level by grade is indicated
	• Not all titles receive positive recommendations
Strengths	• Emphasis on nonprint materials
	• Includes materials written for adults if suitable for younger audience
	• Subject index fiction entries group titles together by subject
	• Introduction outlines evaluative criteria used for items included
Weaknesses	• Titles are old; may not reflect current drug information and attitudes
	• Does not address AIDS and drug use
	• Some current drug terms, such as *crack*, are not indexed

	Child Study Association of America. Book Review Committee. *Recommended Reading About Children and Family Life.* New York: Child Study Association of America, 1969.
Content Synopsis	Designed to provide information sources for parents and persons working in mental health education, this resource addresses the following topics: marriage and family; child development; sex education; physical and emotional disability; school and learning; mental health education; and social problems and family. One chapter, "Children's Books about Special Situations," covers topics pertinent to children's bibliotherapy: hospitalization; death; sibling rivalry; new baby; adoption; foster kids; physical disabilities; divorce; stepfamilies; unstable parents; moving; prejudice and understanding.
Age Levels (as specified in the reference book)	Most titles are for adults. One section is devoted exclusively to children's books, for children aged 4 to 14 years.
Indexes	One index: author/title
Content Parameters	• Titles published prior to 1969

Annotations	• Concise plot summaries that focus on the children or on family life, with suggested age ranges
Strengths	• Age range selected for each title. Does not use predetermined age ranges
Weaknesses	• Recommended titles published prior to 1969 • Language dated (e.g., Negro, retarded)

Cuddigan, Maureen, and Mary Beth Hanson. *Growing Pains: Helping Children Deal with Everyday Problems Through Reading.* Chicago: American Library Association, 1988.

Content Synopsis	Written by a children's librarian and a nurse practitioner, this source identifies quality children's books that focus on themes such as behavior, child abuse, neglect, safety issues, self-concept, and sexual equality. Some themes specifically address emotional adjustment and development issues, such as nighttime fears, anger, or moving. Each chapter has an introduction discussing how that topic relates to children, followed by an annotated bibliography of recommended titles arranged in subtopics.
Age Levels (as specified in the reference book)	Children (scanning entries show most titles for ages 5 through 10)
Indexes	Two indexes: author/title, subject
Content Parameters	• Children's books; most published between 1976 and 1986
Annotations	• Plot summaries emphasize the pertinent theme of the section, such as making friends
Strengths	• Emphasis on quality children's books • Authors read each title included • Introduction emphasizes need for adults to select and preread the titles • Includes chapters on hospitalization, health care, and illness; safety issues; and understanding society • Introduction provides good background material and suggested uses • A few recommended titles at the end of each chapter

	• Includes a few informational books
	• Some titles present positive interactions and relationships—not all negative
Weaknesses	• Titles seem mostly for children under 10 years of age
	• Indicates interest level but not reading level for titles
	• Older titles; though still relevant, most are more than 10 years old
	• Annotations adequate, but do not always capture what is really happening in the book

Dreyer, Sharon Spredemann. *The Best of Bookfinder: A Guide to Children's Literature About Interests and Concerns of Youth Aged 2–18.* Circle Pines, MN: American Guidance Service, 1992.

Content Synopsis	Designed to assist parents, counselors, teachers, librarians, psychologists, and psychiatrists in identifying books that can help children cope with life's challenges, this reference work describes and categorizes 676 children's books according to more than 450 psychological, behavioral, and developmental topics pertinent to children and adolescents. Following an overview of bibliotherapy, the introduction discusses how *Bookfinder* was developed and gives advice on how to use the source. Annotations are arranged alphabetically by author. Dreyer has a master's degree in education.
Age Levels (as specified in the reference book)	2 to 18 years
Indexes	Three indexes: subject, author, title
Content Parameters	• Titles published primarily during 1970s and 1980s; some earlier titles included
	• Emphasis on fiction titles
	• Titles in print at time of this publication
	• Attempts to include quality titles with realistic characters and problem resolution without didacticism
Annotations	• Lengthy paragraphs give a detailed synopsis of the book's plot
	• Discusses each title's strengths and weaknesses, as well as potential uses

- Indicates reading-level range, appropriate subject headings, and/or primary and secondary themes
- Also gives other forms of publication, such as filmstrips, paperbound editions, tapes, films, records, and materials for blind or other physically disabled people

Strengths

- Selections represent the best books from *Bookfinders* 1–3 (works published prior to 1983)
- Includes annotated list of recommended book selection aids and a bibliography of readings on bibliotherapy
- Covers wide range of bibliotherapy-relevant topics, including the following sample subject headings: abandonment, aggression, courage, death, emotional deprivation, fear, friendship, gender role identity, inferiority, jealousy, loyalty, mental illness, nightmares, peer relationships, prejudice, prostitution, rape, resourcefulness, self-esteem, sex, siblings, stealing, suicide, tantrums, trust, values, visual impairment, weight control, and women's rights

Weaknesses

- Lacks the physically flexible index of early editions; earlier editions were formatted as two books within one casing, with the index volume at the top and annotations at the bottom. This format enabled the user to browse through the annotations and consult the index without flipping back and forth between the two

Fassler, Joan. *Helping Children Cope.* New York: Free Press, 1978.

Content Synopsis

This source serves as a resource of titles to be used for discussion with children in helping them deal with stressful experiences. Each chapter focuses on one of five themes: death; separation experiences; hospitalization and illness; lifestyle changes; and other potentially stress-producing situations. At the end of each chapter, there is a list of references to the professional literature and a bibliography of the juvenile books covered. The author is affiliated with the Yale University Child Study Center.

Age Levels (as specified in the reference book)

Primarily 4 to 8 years old; some books for older children

Indexes	Two indexes: Juvenile Book Authors, general
Content Parameters	• Books included are those that author has used for specific situations
	• Most titles published during the 1960s and 1970s; some titles published during the 1940s and 1950s
Annotations	• Embedded in text under topical subheadings
	• Some annotations give only a plot summary; others discuss the book at length and provide suggested questions for discussion
Strengths	• Emphasis on ways to discuss the issues raised by the books with children
	• Explores each topic from various angles and perspectives
	• Includes examples of nonrecommended titles and describes why those titles are poor selections
Weaknesses	• No specific reading or grade levels are indicated for titles

Field, Carolyn W., and Jaqueline Shachter Weiss. *Values in Selected Children's Books of Fiction and Fantasy.* Hamden, CT: Library Professional Publication, 1987.

Content Synopsis	This practical guide to fiction and fantasy is a selection of titles that emphasize positive values for children, as well as titles that help children to develop their own standards. Containing 142 books for early years, 213 books for middle years, and 358 books for later years, the chapters cover the following values: cooperation; courage; friendship and love of animals; friendship and love of people; humaneness; ingenuity; loyalty; maturing; responsibility; and self-respect.
Age Levels (as specified in the reference book)	Preschool to grade 8
Indexes	Two indexes: title, author
Content Parameters	• Titles published or distributed in United States from 1930 to 1984, with an emphasis on recent titles
	• Fiction titles

Annotations	• Plot summaries embedded in text, which may include a quotation from the book itself to illustrate the particular value being addressed
	• Titles grouped within chapter by age range
	• No evaluative comments
Strengths	• Some out-of-print books included
	• All titles recommended
Weaknesses	• Annotations do not include evaluative or analytical comments

Friedberg, Joan Brest, June B. Mullins, and Adelaide Weir Sukiennik. *Accept Me As I Am: Best Books of Juvenile Nonfiction on Impairments and Disabilities.* New York: R. R. Bowker, 1985.

Content Synopsis	This source aims to promote understanding of and tolerance for the disabled through a selective list of nonfiction titles that portray the experiences of people with disabilities or impairments in a realistic, perceptive, and sensitive manner. Nonfiction categories covered include: biography, autobiography, concept, and information books about people who are disabled. Following historical and background information, annotations in chapters 5 to 8 are arranged in broad, disability categories: physical, sensory, cognitive, and behavior problems and multiple or severe and various disabilities. Subcategories address specific impairments.
Age Levels (as specified in the reference book)	Ages 2 to 17 years; some titles appropriate for adults
Indexes	Three indexes: author, title, subject
Content Parameters	• Nonfiction titles published before 1984
Annotations	• Plot summaries, followed by a brief, critical analysis of literary and disability elements
	• Indicates reading level by grade and lists the disability
	• Often recommends what kind of readers would enjoy or benefit from each title
Strengths	• Includes a professional bibliography of books for teachers and librarians
	• Works included are selected for quality
	• Covers a wide variety of disabilities, including emotional disturbances

Weaknesses	• Most titles seem to be for older readers, grades 7 to 12

Gillespie, John T., and Corinne J. Naden. *Juniorplots 3: A Book Talk Guide for Use with Readers Ages 12–16.* New York: R. R. Bowker, 1987.

——. *Seniorplots: A Book Talk Guide for Use with Readers Ages 15–18.* New York: R. R. Bowker, 1989.

Content Synopsis	Both resources suggest titles to be used for booktalks and each resource also serves as a general reading guidance tool. Highlighting 80 titles each, these sources identify books that are likely to appeal to young people as well as books that have value in a variety of situations. Sample chapter headings include: teenage life and concerns; adventures and mystery; science fiction and fantasy; historical fiction; sports fiction; biography and true adventure; guidance and health; and the world around us.
Age Levels (as specified in the reference book)	*Juniorplots*: 12 to 16 years *Seniorplots*: 15 to 18 years
Indexes	Three indexes: author, title, subject
Content Parameters	• Both reference books include titles published primarily in the 1980s
Annotations	• After a brief introduction, lengthy plot summaries detail each book's content • Additional sections discuss themes in the book, possible selections for booktalking, and suggest other titles that address similar themes • Also includes citations for book reviews and sources of further information about the author
Strengths	• Includes novels written for adult audience (*Seniorplots*) • Subject index allows access to suitable bibliotherapeutic topics, such as suicide, sexual abuse, alcoholism, mothers and sisters, child abuse, death and dying, courage, divorce, families, and abortion • Covers major genres

- Titles included were recommended for purchase from several standard bibliographies and reviewing sources
- Additional titles are suggested for same themes
- Includes some nonfiction

Weaknesses

- Only limited number of titles are covered in depth

Gillis, Ruth J. *Children's Books for Times of Stress: An Annotated Bibliography.* Bloomington: Indiana University Press, 1978.

Content Synopsis

This source aims to provide books for young children that will help them to cope with a range of emotionally stressful situations. The 261 annotations are arranged alphabetically under broad subject headings: emotions, behavior, family, difficult situations, new situations, self-concept, and friendship. Subheadings, such as jealousy, teasing, extended family, illness, need for eyeglasses, shyness, and loneliness, further divide each category. A list of subject headings and subheadings used, as well as a key to review sources, are also included. The author is a school librarian at University Elementary School.

Age Levels (as specified in the reference book)

Preschool to 9 years

Indexes

Three indexes: title, author, illustrator

Content Parameters

- Books published primarily from 1960 to 1976
- Individual titles had to be located in standard professional review source to be included in this bibliography

Annotations

- Concise plot summaries, sometimes enhanced by evaluative comments
- Includes assigned subject headings and indicates the review source

Strengths

- Annotations reproduced under each relevant subheading/heading
- Titles selected on basis of literary quality, with some exceptions if the title was deemed critical for providing material in a needed area
- Each book critically examined by author
- Wide range of emotional aspects covered, such as death, divorce, hospitalization, shyness, friendship, love, happiness, and bravery

Weaknesses	• Typeface difficult to read • Titles are not assigned a specific reading or age level

Horner, Catherine Townsend. *The Single-Parent Family in Children's Books: An Annotated Bibliography.* 2d ed. Metuchen, NJ: Scarecrow Press, 1988.

Content Synopsis	This collection of nonselective, fiction and nonfiction titles represents the single-parent family in its various manifestations. The introduction traces the history of single-parent representation in children's fiction and notes that since 1980, novels with single-parent families present a serious and often realistic portrayal of the situation. An annotated bibliography is arranged by the following categories: divorce, desertion, separation; widowhood; unwed mothers; orphans, wards of court with single guardian; protracted absence of one parent (from a two-parent home); and indeterminate cause.
Age Levels (as specified in the reference book)	Grades K to 10
Indexes	Two indexes: title (which includes brief plot synopses), author/subject
Content Parameters	• Fiction titles published between 1965 and 1986 • Selections limited to books available from Santa Clara County, California, public libraries during research period
Annotations	• Descriptive plot summaries, with an emphasis on value for a single-parent book collection • Indicates reading level and gives a rating that ranges from "not recommended" to "highest recommendation" • Some nonfiction annotations are in a separate section and indicate content summary and reading level
Strengths	• Title index entries include a short plot summary for ready reference referral • Only highly recommended nonfiction books included • Includes some "classics" published before 1965

Weaknesses	• Nonfiction titles not accessible through indexes
	• Because titles receive ratings instead of evaluative comments, can be difficult to identify specific reasons for the rating

Hyde, Margaret O. *Sexual Abuse: Let's Talk About It.* Rev. ed. Philadelphia: Westminster Press, 1987.

Content Synopsis	Designed to educate people about sexual abuse, with an emphasis on protection, prevention, and treatment, the eight chapters in this source cover topics ranging from sexual abuse, good and bad touching, and who are the offenders to how to prevent sexual abuse. Case studies are used throughout to add "real-world" elements and interest. Hyde is both a teacher and an author of children's informational books.
Age Levels (as specified in the reference book)	Preschool to senior high school
Indexes	One index: title/author/subject
Content Parameters	• Bibliography includes only 21 titles of books and audiovisual materials, all of which were published between 1979 and 1986
Annotations	• None
Strengths	• Titles specifically address sexual abuse of children
	• Includes both fiction and nonfiction
Weaknesses	• Limited number of titles
	• More of an informational book than a reference book

Miller-Lachmann, Lyn. *Our Family, Our Friends, Our World: An Annotated Guide to Significant Multicultural Books for Children and Teenagers.* New Providence, NJ: R. R. Bowker, 1992.

Content Synopsis	This source provides an annotated list of both fiction and nonfiction multicultural books, with an emphasis on cultural diversity within geographical world regions. Approximately 1,000 entries, both national and international in scope, are arranged geographically; titles are also organized by grade level within each chapter. The work was compiled by 21 contributors, most of whom are children's services librarians and school media specialists but who also include teachers, educational consultants, academicians, and children's literature authors.

Age Levels (as specified in the reference book)	Preschool to grade 12
Indexes	Three indexes: author, title/series, subject. Rich in multicultural titles, the subject index can be used to identify titles most appropriate to bibliotherapy, such as on family problems, adoption, blindness, or self-esteem.
Content Parameters	• Fiction and nonfiction published between 1970 and 1990 in the United States and Canada
Annotations	• Concise content/plot summaries followed by evaluative commentary • Evaluates text and illustration or photograph quality
Strengths	• Chapters compiled by a subject specialist for that area • Includes an annotated appendix of professional sources to be used by teachers/librarians as companion works for each chapter, such as films, videos, and music • Fully and carefully explains guidelines for inclusion or exclusion of specific titles • Contains a history of the publishing of multicultural titles • Includes both recommended and not-recommended titles so users can compare
Weaknesses	• None identified

Polette, Nancy. *Books and Real Life: A Guide for Gifted Students and Teachers.* Jefferson, NC: McFarland, 1984.

Content Synopsis	The author, a professor of education at Lindenwood Colleges, St. Charles, Missouri, and an author of children's books, has compiled a resource to help adults identify titles for gifted children to help these young people cope with life. Realistic fiction addresses how to deal with such problems as violence, fear, death, anger, divorce, family relationships, rejection, handicaps, friendship, and old age. The section of titles for preschool and primary-school students covers relationships, events, values, and feelings; the section of junior novels includes decision making, problem solving, and forecasting.

Age Levels (as specified in the reference book)	Preschool to high school
Indexes	One index: subject
Content Parameters	• Most titles published in the 1970s; includes only a few titles published in the early 1980s
Annotations	• Concise plot summaries followed by suggested activities and questions to stimulate discussion
Strengths	• Suggested questions for discussion • Titles selected use realistic and psychologically sound approaches to dealing with the problems presented
Weaknesses	• Does not suggest reading levels for each title • Organization of junior novels chapter is confusing • Not all titles in junior novels section are annotated

	Reading Ladders for Human Relations. 6th ed. Edited by Eileen Tway. Washington, DC: American Council on Education, 1981.
Content Synopsis	This source aims to provide books of good literary quality that promote sensitivity in human relations. Fiction, nonfiction, and poetry titles are arranged under five major categories: Growing into Self; Relating to Wide Individual Differences; Interacting in Groups; Appreciating Different Cultures; and Coping in a Changing World. Eileen Tway is the Chair of the National Council of Teachers of English (NCTE) Committee on Reading Ladders for Human Relations, a committee composed of both teachers and librarians.
Age Levels (as specified in the reference book)	Preschool to high school
Indexes	Two indexes: author, title
Content Parameters	Primarily books printed since fifth edition (1972)
Annotations	• Very precise plot summaries • Occasional evaluative comments
Strengths	• Selection criteria outlined in introduction • Some titles cross-referenced between sections • Chapters conclude with a list of professional references

	• Includes fiction and nonfiction • Each chapter has an introduction written by the team that compiled those titles
Weaknesses	• Not all annotations are evaluative • Many titles published in the 1970s • No subject index

	Robertson, Debra E. J. *Portraying Persons with Disabilities: An Annotated Bibliography of Fiction for Children and Teenagers.* 3d ed. New Providence, NJ: R. R. Bowker, 1992.
Content Synopsis	Written by a librarian who is handicapped, this source is designed to provide a selection of titles that portray characters with a range of different emotional and physical disabilities or impairments. Following introductory and background comments, chapters 4 through 7 present titles that address physical problems, sensory problems, cognitive and behavior problems, and multiple/severe and various disabilities.
Age Levels (as specified in the reference book)	Preschool to grade 12
Indexes	Three indexes: author, title, subject
Content Parameters	• Fiction titles published between 1982 and 1991
Annotations	• Lengthy plot summaries, with emphasis on the subject disability or impairment, followed by critical content analysis • Entries indicate a reading-level range and identify the disability at the top
Strengths	• Includes professional bibliography • Annotations grouped by broad disability categories • Full annotations not given for seriously flawed titles • Chapter 1 emphasizes pertinent titles from *Notes from a Different Drummer: A Guide to Juvenile Fiction Portraying the Handicapped* by Barbara H. Baskin and Karen H. Harris (New York: R. R. Bowker, 1977) and *More Notes from a Different Drummer: A Guide to Juvenile Fiction Portraying the Handicapped* by Barbara H. Baskin and Karen H. Harris (New York: R. R. Bowker, 1984) (the latter is described here)

Weaknesses	• Most titles for middle to older readers

Spirt, Diana L. *Introducing Bookplots 3: A Book Talk Guide for Use with Readers Ages 8–12.* New York: R. R. Bowker, 1988.

Content Synopsis	This source serves as a reading guidance and book-talk reference tool for librarians and other adults who work to stimulate reading interest among middle-graders. Each chapter contains nine titles that reflect the developmental goals of getting along in the family, making friends, developing values, understanding physical and emotional problems, forming a view of the world, respecting living creatures, understanding social problems, identifying adult roles, and appreciating books. The author is emeritus professor of children's books and materials, Palmer School of Library and Information Science, Long Island University.
Age Levels (as specified in the reference book)	Ages 8 to 12
Indexes	Three indexes: biographical, title/author/illustrator, subject
Content Parameters	• Titles published between 1979 and 1986
Annotations	• Detailed, extensive plot summaries begin with information about the author • Includes discussion of themes (thematic analysis), specific suggestions for booktalks or discussion, and related sections on book materials (fiction, nonfiction, and audiovisual materials)
Strengths	• Titles listed within each chapter by range of difficulty for middle-graders • Related materials recommended for each title often include filmstrips, videos, and recordings, as well as books • End of each chapter contains a list of unannotated titles (print and nonprint) on the same topic or theme • Titles are recommended by at least three reputable reviewing sources and were read by author • Includes a directory of audiovisual publishers and distributors
Weaknesses	• Primarily fiction titles

Sutherland, Zena, Betsy Hearne, and Roger Sutton.
The Best in Children's Books: The University of Chicago Guide to Children's Literature, 1985–1990. Chicago: University of Chicago Press, 1991.

Content Synopsis	Reviewed originally in the *Bulletin of the Center for Children's Books* between 1985 and 1990, these titles represent the best American and British fiction and nonfiction. All entries received a recommended rating. A section called "Suggestions for Using this Book" outlines the criteria for the indexes. Sutherland is a professor emeritus in the Graduate Library School at the University of Chicago and a former editor of the *Bulletin of the Center for Children's Books*. Hearne is the editor and Sutton is the executive editor of the *Bulletin*.
Age Levels (as specified in the reference book)	Six months to grade 10; indicated both in years and grade levels
Indexes	Six indexes: title, developmental values, curricular use, reading level, subject, and type of literature
Content Parameters	• Only American and British fiction and non-fiction that received recommended ratings in the University of Chicago's *Bulletin of the Center for Children's Books* • All titles published between 1985 and 1990
Annotations	• Brief plot or content summaries embedded in the critical evaluation
Strengths	• Introduction covers criteria for evaluating and identifying a good children's book • Reading levels are given in ranges (not predetermined, but varying to meet the specifics of each title) • Several useful indexes, most specifically the developmental values index • Titles selected for literary quality
Weaknesses	• Brief evaluations

Wilkin, Binnie Tate. *Survival Themes in Fiction for Children and Young People.* 2nd ed. Metuchen, NJ: Scarecrow Press, 1993.

Content Synopsis	This source seeks to provide a collection of contemporary, realistic children's fiction titles that explore issues

of human existence and survival. In addition, selected books encourage readers to ask the right questions—a skill that may be a critical survival skill for today's youth. Titles, carefully selected for their literary quality, explore issues such as loneliness, peer pressure, or religion that may cause problems for children or young adults in their daily lives. The author is a consultant in library services with an emphasis on public libraries and children's services. Her previous positions include: school librarian, children's librarian, minority services coordinator for the Los Angeles County Public Library, and teacher at the University of California at Berkeley, UCLA, and University of Wisconsin–Milwaukee library schools.

Age Levels (as specified in the reference book)	Preschool to high school
Indexes	Three indexes: author, title, illustrator
Content Parameters	• Books published primarily in the 1980s
Annotations	• Plot summaries and evaluative comments stress the relationship between the title and the survival theme
	• Some annotations are very brief and reveal little about the plot
Strengths	• Emphasis placed on titles that show characters' introspection and growth; cover social development and interaction; depict varied personality types and cultures; and provide different perspectives on historical, political, and environmental issues
	• Covers children's experiences of war
	• Suggests selected audiovisual sources for each chapter's theme and notes which titles should be used in conjunction with audiovisual material
	• The "Sources and Notes" section, a selectively annotated list of nonfiction and fiction titles, includes many titles about children's literature
	• Suggests programming activities for each section
Weaknesses	• Titles for younger readers are not evaluated as extensively as titles for older readers—sometimes not at all
	• Annotation length varies for all age ranges

	Zivrin, Stephanie. *The Best Years of Their Lives: A Resource Guide for Teenagers in Crisis.* Chicago: American Library Association, 1992.
Content Synopsis	This source is a selective guide primarily to nonfiction, self-help books geared to an adolescent audience and their specific concerns and problems. Nine chapters list self-help fiction, nonfiction, and videos on the following topics: family relationships; attitudes toward school; self-image; substance abuse; rape, incest, and physical violence; health issues, including stress, anorexia, and depression; sexuality; pregnancy and parenting; and death, including teen suicide as well as the death of family and friends. The author is a former high school teacher and public librarian, and was an associate editor for *Booklist* at the time of publication.
Age Levels (as specified in the reference book	Adolescents aged 12 to 18 (some titles suggested for (age 10+)
Indexes	Two indexes: author/title, subject
Content Parameters	• More nonfiction than fiction titles • Titles published after 1986 • Emphasis on readily available materials (such as those from major publishers)
Annotations	• Nonfiction annotations include content summary, evaluation, and suggested age levels • Fiction annotations include age levels and plot summary, but no evaluative comments
Strengths	• Includes a filmography of recommended videos, both documentaries and dramatizations, released primarily during the late 1980s to early 1990s. The filmography was compiled by the nonprint materials assistant editor of *Booklist*. Titles cover the same subjects addressed in the bibliography • Includes interviews with several contributing authors
Weaknesses	• Annotations less extensive for fiction than nonfiction titles, and consist only of plot summaries

REFERENCES

Lee, Lauren K., ed. 1994. *Elementary School Library Collection: A Guide to Books and Other Media*. 19th ed. Williamsport, PA: Brodart.

Smith, Brenda, and Juliette Yaakov, eds. 1992. *Senior High School Library Catalog*. 14th ed. New York: H. W. Wilson.

Yaakov, Juliette, ed. 1990. *Junior High School Library Catalog*. 6th ed. New York: H. W. Wilson.

———. 1991. *Children's Catalog*. 16th ed. New York: H. W. Wilson.

8 Building a Bibliotherapy Program

If a single lesson could be drawn from the accumulated research on child therapy, it would be this: Results of therapy are generally ineffective when the therapy is haphazard and undirected (Rose and Edelson 1987). While assuming that this is also true of bibliotherapy programs, we use this chapter to describe a nine-step procedure for leaders to use in planning systematic bibliotherapy programs. The steps are detailed as a nine-question checklist to be completed as effective bibliotherapy programs proceed.

The nine questions are these:

1. Which and how many children and youth will this bibliotherapy program serve?

2. If successful, what will the program accomplish for those participants?

3. Which professionals should be responsible for planning, implementing, and monitoring this bibliotherapy program?

4. If more than one professional is responsible for the bibliotherapy program, what kind of working relationship do they need to support the program adequately? What will they do to support that relationship?

5. What type of media, and which selections, will best match the participants and purpose of this bibliotherapy program?

6. What activities will be used to reinforce the participants' comprehension
of the selections? Which activities maximize the chances that participants
will actually apply the materials' lessons to their own lives?

7. Who will be responsible for monitoring participants' responses to the media, to ensure that they are not unduly stressed or harmed by topics and
the manner in which the topics are raised? If there is evidence that one or
more participants require more extensive child therapy, who will ensure
that they are referred to an alternative program of therapy? Where will
they be referred for more extensive child therapy services?

8. If one or more participants are youths with serious emotional disturbances,
who will extend the program into a comprehensive program of clinical bibliotherapy? How will that person establish an action plan to prompt the youths
to apply the selection's lessons to their own lives? How will that plan be moni-
tored? Who will review and revise the plan with the children, and how?

9. Did the program achieve its purpose?

As each of the questions is answered, in turn, a carefully planned program of bibliotherapy
will emerge.

1. WHICH YOUTH TO SERVE

Ultimately, the intent of any program of bibliotherapy is to improve the quality of life for youth in the community. Because these children and adolescents represent a diverse group of individuals, it is important to decide in advance who
among them will be the target of a program. At a minimum, three characteristics
should be used to predefine the participants in any bibliotherapy program: the degree of socioemotional distress or disturbance that the program can accommodate,
the age range that the program will serve, and the interests that the program will
meet. Variations in any of these three can significantly alter the nature of program
activities, the selection of program materials, and the requirements for particular
kinds of professional expertise.

Level of Socioemotional Distress

Chapter 3 describes ranges of socioemotional distress in greater detail for
three groups of youth: children with significant socioemotional disturbances, those
who are socially vulnerable and at risk for poor social and emotional outcomes,
and developmentally typical children coping with disturbing but common difficulties of growing up. If a bibliotherapy program is targeted toward either of the first
two groups, plans should be made to secure reliable participation and support from
a mental health professional. These professionals have the skills to more clearly
identify the young persons' problems and help them work toward solutions. Alternatively, if the program will target developmentally typical children, the adult
mentorship it will require is probably adequately served by a community's child librarians and media specialists, given their training in child and adolescent development and the rapport they have established with their young patrons.

Age of Participants

The age of youth participating in a program has obvious implications for the readability, thematic maturity, and the social lessons of media selected for the program. Other constraints imposed by age are less obvious. Chapter 2 describes developmental differences in children's ability to solve social problems, set personal goals, and understand the social perspective of others. Children in whom these skills are just emerging will need extensive adult support in picking out the lessons from a book, understanding a book's applicability to their own lives, or recognizing the needs and motivations of fictional characters. Adolescents, because they are generally well advanced in all of these interpersonal skills, are more independent in applying a book to their own lives. Small differences in these abilities are advantageous for a group discussion, because children reasoning at more sophisticated levels benefit from opportunities to explain a book's principles to their less sophisticated peers, and their explanations tend to be more developmentally appropriate than those offered by adults. However, it is generally unwise to plan a program of bibliotherapy for participants whose ages span more than three years because, when ages differ too much, the discrepancies in understanding may be too large, difficult, or tedious for the children to overcome.

Interests

Differences in children's interests are just as important to consider. Bibliotherapy programs are strengthened by the enticement of reading an exciting book or watching a moving film. However, when the selected materials attempt to span too broad a range of interests, the group may lose its attraction. Subsequently, too much energy of the adult leader will be preoccupied with managing irritating and disruptive behaviors and too little spent in reflective guidance about the book. Motivational differences can present special problems in cases where a program of bibliotherapy is planned around a single problem, such as stepfamilies or giftedness. A common mistake is to assume that all children having the problem will be interested in reading about and discussing it. In such cases, it is wise to describe the topic of the group to potential participants and allow them to voluntarily choose to participate.

2. PURPOSES OF THE PROGRAM

Seven purposes addressed through bibliotherapy programs were described in chapter 2. These were: fostering personal insight, triggering emotional catharsis, assisting with solving problems, altering the ways in which children act, promoting satisfying relationships with peers, providing information about shared problems, and recreation. Depending upon which purposes are targeted by a particular program of bibliotherapy, different plans will be made for staffing the program and different activities will be used to foster children's comprehension.

When programs intend to prompt intense emotional responses in the participating youth, wisdom dictates that a mental health professional contribute to the program's planning and management. Not only do these specialists have special knowledge about ways to foster emotional engagement, but they are also alert to the signs that a child's emotional response is too intense and unhelpful. The contributions of mental health professionals will also be useful for programs that work to change children's actual behaviors. Behavior change strategies are well developed within the mental health professions, and these specialists are alert to signs that a behavior change program has to be adjusted so as to continue to be effective.

Alternatively, competence in fostering insight, directing problem-solving activities, and providing opportunities for peer interactions are well within the expertise of most children's librarians. Moreover, it could be argued that librarians and media specialists have special abilities in directing children to specific sources of information and in recognizing and fostering recreation through books and media.

3. DECIDING UPON STAFFING

Once decisions have been made about the program's purposes and targeted participants, it is possible to determine whether the program is essentially one of developmental or clinical bibliotherapy. This decision, then, determines who should share responsibility for planning, implementation, and evaluation. Program staffing decisions should be based on the match between the professional's skills and the needs of the program.

When the program being planned is clearly one of developmental bibliotherapy, the children being targeted will be those with developmentally typical problems, and the purposes defined for the program will not involve emotional catharsis or extensive behavioral change. For such developmental programs, chapter 4 describes the special skills that the librarian or media specialist has to contribute. Librarians and media specialists are trained professionals with backgrounds in child and adolescent development and cognitive psychology. They usually encounter and work with young people daily. This type of contact gives librarians and media specialists access to young people and the opportunity to build mentoring relationships with them. Moreover, as discussed in chapter 4, librarians and media specialists are experts in the area of children's or young adult materials. Their highly developed skill in identifying and locating books or other materials on specific topics, and in matching these materials to specific young individuals, is unique to the library profession and an invaluable contribution to bibliotherapy. Also, librarians and media specialists are very good at discussing books, videos, and other materials with young people.

When the program will target children or adolescents facing a more difficult problem, and the purposes of the program are clearly aligned with those of a child therapy regimen, clinical bibliotherapy may be appropriate. For such a program, a trained mental health professional should be involved. These professionals have the skills needed to identify the child's most pressing problem and then plan a program of therapeutic services that helps the young person develop strategies for coping with or solving the problem. These specialized skills make it possible for them to extend a program of bibliotherapy into a broader regimen of child therapy, as described more fully in chapter 5. Moreover, as co-leaders of a bibliotherapy discussion, mental health specialists are prepared to note and intervene when vulnerable children have unhelpful reactions to a book or activity. Finally, mental health specialists know how to link a bibliotherapy program into a community's mental health system, so that vulnerable children can be easily referred for more assistance should that become necessary.

From this discussion, it should be obvious that both sets of professionals have skills in establishing rapport with young people and in discussing materials with them. At the same time, both sets of professionals have specialized training that enables them to make unique contributions. Librarians and media specialists know books and other materials and are able to match suitable titles to specific children. Mental health professionals know how to recognize and treat the more serious disturbances young people may suffer. In many cases, then, library professionals and mental health professionals can potentially offer young people stronger, more effective bibliotherapy experiences by working together than by working separately.

4. CREATING PROFESSIONAL TEAMS

Increasingly, experts in professional relationships have come to understand that the creation of effective professional teams presents special challenges as well as special opportunities (Conoley and Conoley 1992). Professional teams will be most effective when:

- All members of the team are included, from the beginning, in the planning and decision making for a program of bibliotherapy
- The various team members share an agreed-upon purpose for the program
- The team members share information readily and frankly throughout the program
- The individualized contribution of each team member is synchronized with that person's special skills and knowledge
- The members of the team are mutually supportive of each other's efforts.

These kinds of professional teams emerge from relationships that are carefully planned and mutually supported. To clarify, table 8.1 describes three variations on two professional teams that might support a bibliotherapy program, and the optimal ways for each member of the team to act within the relationship. *Cooperative teams* are those in which each professional is responsible for a distinct program of service to the same group of children, but each member shares information about the other's services and both work to minimize conflicts and contradictions. *Consultative teams* are those in which one professional retains the essential responsibility for planning, implementing, and evaluating a bibliotherapy program, but relies on the assistance of the other in the domains in which that professional is expert. *Collaborative teams* are those in which both professionals share responsibility for the bibliotherapy program, relying on each other's expertise in domains in which they are less experienced.

Once two or more professionals have decided to provide a bibliotherapy program as a team, an important first step is to determine the kind of team within which they will work. That decision determines how the subsequent planning and implementation of the program will proceed. When teams are working consultatively or collaboratively, it will be important to determine what special skills and talents each member brings to the team. Assistance in making that determination can be found in chapters 4 and 5, with the first describing some special competencies of librarians and media specialists and the latter describing the special competencies of mental health professionals.

Table 8.1. Types of Professional Teams

Type of Team	Professional 1	Professional 2	When This Type Is Appropriate
Cooperative	Assume primary responsibility for planning, implementing, and monitoring one's own services. Inform Professional 2 about one's own services, which children they serve, and the purposes of the services. Reinforce purposes of Professional 2's services as opportunities arise.	Assume primary responsibility for planning, implementing, and monitoring one's own services. Inform Professional 1 about one's own services, which children they serve, and the purposes of the services. Reinforce purposes of Professional 1's services as opportunities arise.	When two professionals are working with the same groups of children but have very different purposes guiding their services; this kind of team ensures that the services provided by one do not contradict or lessen the impact of services offered by the other.
Consultative	Assume primary responsibility for planning, implementing, and monitoring one's own services. Inform Professional 2 about one's own services, which children they serve, and the purposes of the services. Request information and assistance from Professional 2 for skills and knowledge in which he or she is more expert. Incorporate the knowledge and skills gained from Professional 2 into one's own services.	Attend to Professional 1's explanation of the services he or she offers. Provide information and assistance to Professional 1 as one's own expertise supports those services. Check back with Professional 1 periodically to offer additional information and assistance, as appropriate.	When one professional's working conditions make it impossible to assume shared responsibility for a bibliotherapy program; this kind of team makes it possible for the principal professional to benefit from the special expertise of the consulting professional.
Collaborative	Include Professional 2 in all planning, implementation, and evaluation of the program, including the early stages of program planning when shared purposes and participants are selected. Articulate a plan for the bibliotherapy program that incorporates Professional 2's ideas and skills as well as one's own. Contribute one's own skills to the bibiotherapy program as determined by the plan. Support the ongoing relationship with Professional 2 by listening carefully to that person's comments, staying open to new ideas that he or she contributes, and continuing to share decision making with that person.	Include Professional 1 in all planning, implementation, and evaluation of the program, including the early stages of program planning when shared purposes and participants are selected. Articulate a plan for the bibliotherapy program that incorporates Professional 1's ideas and skills as well as one's own. Contribute one's own skills to the bibliotherapy program as determined by the plan. Support the ongoing relationship with Professional 1 by listening carefully to that person's comments, staying open to new ideas that he or she contributes, and continuing to share decision making with that person.	When both professionals are willing to share responsibilities of the program; this kind of team makes it possible for the expertise of both to be fully utilized within the program.

One final word of warning is necessary. In work relationships, it is all too easy for one profession to hold stereotypic views of the competencies of other professions—views that are rooted in the other profession's traditions, historical experiences, or standards of training. On occasion, these professional reputations can be overgeneralizations that fail to give credit to the other professional for his or her unique talents. It is important to remember that competence is a characteristic of a person, not a profession, and that effective professional relationships are fostered one person at a time.

5. SELECTING APPROPRIATE MEDIA

The selection of suitable books and films for children and adolescents is a special skill of librarians and media specialists. The use of topical bibliographies to support this selection is described more fully in chapter 7. Still, these resources are not entirely sufficient to support good book and film selection by bibliotherapy leaders who are not trained in the evaluation of children's literature. In addition to locating books on the correct topic, and ensuring that the materials' treatment of that topic is both accurate and sensitive, materials selection requires a comprehensive examination of the plot, characterization, and writing style used in the book. Likewise, selection of films and videos requires these skills as well as careful examination of the implications inherent in the film's visual images. These selection skills, as practiced by librarians and media specialists, are described in more detail in chapter 4.

6. PLANNING COMPREHENSION ACTIVITIES

The activities that a program uses to reinforce the lessons of a book or film are critically important determinants of whether the program's purpose is served. Chapter 2 explains alternative times and formats that comprehension activities can take, and the annotated bibliography in appendix A identifies several professional references that provide alternative ideas for activities. Activities should be selected because they match the program's purpose, are developmentally appropriate for the age range of the program's participants, and are likely to be interesting so as to prompt active engagement by the participants.

The match between activities and a program's purposes may be the most difficult to anticipate. Table 8.2 describes this match in more detail and provides examples of activities exemplifying each purpose. In practice, the importance of purpose in choosing activities is often overlooked; as a consequence, programs may miss opportunities to reinforce the lessons they believe most important for the reader.

Secondarily, the developmental demands of different activities should be carefully evaluated. For example, their limited role-taking skills make it difficult for young, elementary-school-age children to analyze the conflicting motivations or feelings of a fictional character. Early adolescents may not have mastered abstract reasoning skills sufficiently to create alternative, hypothetical endings of a book. Young children may find it difficult to apply examples from the books to their own lives unless the situations between the two are virtually identical. Some guidance in examining these developmental constraints can be found in chapter 2.

Table 8.2. Matching Comprehension Activities to Purposes of Bibliotherapy Programs

Purpose of the Program	Activities Required
Fostering personal insight	Activities that draw attention to the commonalities between the fictional characters and the readers. E.g., Pardeck (1989) suggests that children sketch out two story lines—one for the events in the book and a parallel one of their own lives.
Triggering emotional catharsis	Activities that help children and adolescents notice, define, verbalize, and cope with feelings. E.g., Bump (1990) asks adolescents to reflect on the characters they most liked and most disliked before analyzing what features of the characters drew out those emotional responses. Pardeck (1990) suggests that children create "mood collages" to capture the emotional themes of a book.
Assisting with solving problems	Activities that guide children and adolescents through the systematic problem-solving steps of identifying the problem, listing alternative solutions, evaluating the impact of different solutions, and selecting the most appropriate solution. E.g., Pardeck (1989) suggests that children write a different ending for a character in the book, or make a poster listing problem solutions that the fictional characters attempted and highlight the ones that worked for them.
Altering the ways in which children act	Activities that assist children in seeing the connections between the ways in which fictional characters act and their own lives, and that prompt children to plan new ways of behaving. E.g., create a "time capsule" containing the children's written plans to mimic effective behaviors of fictional characters. Return to the time capsule weeks later and report successful plans.
Promoting satisfying relationships with peers	Activities that engage children and adolescents in interactions that are enjoyable and promote new opportunities for interactions. E.g., ask children to work in pairs when role playing, creating book collages, or redesigning book jackets. Suggest that children learn together to play some of the games described in a novel.
Providing information about shared problems	Activities that draw attention to the factual knowledge contained in a book, organizing it, or emphasizing it so that children take notice of it. E.g., Jeon (1992) recommends that the group view films or filmstrips on topics similar to the book; Bump (1990) co-assigns self-help books that explain the dynamics depicted in a piece of literature.
Recreation	Activities that are fun!

Finally, activities should be chosen for their attractiveness and creativity. One important determinant of attractiveness is novelty—when programs employ variations on the same activity repeatedly, the interest of the group will wane quickly and behavior problems will begin to emerge.

7. IMPLEMENTING THE PROGRAM

It is common for bibliotherapy leaders to notice errors in their earlier planning once a program of bibliotherapy has begun, the children are reading, and activities are proceeding. Perhaps the activities were too challenging or too easy for the children that attend, or perhaps the books and media are too difficult to read. It is possible that the children participating in the program are more emotionally vulnerable than had been anticipated. In any case, plans for the bibliotherapy program should be reviewed and fine-tuned throughout the program to correct these errors. Effective revisions will maintain or tighten the program's focus on the essential purposes it attempts to achieve.

A second challenge in program implementation is monitoring the responses of the children in the group. Because the children themselves will not always voice their distress, chapter 6 describes indicators that might become evident if one or more participants are becoming unusually anxious or upset by various aspects of the program. Alternatively, chapter 3 provides additional information about children's socioemotional disturbances, and may be consulted as a quick reference for understanding participants in a group. Even if a program was not initially planned in collaboration with a mental health professional, it could become necessary to confer with such a specialist if children's needs prompt it.

8. EXTENSIONS REQUIRED BY CLINICAL BIBLIOTHERAPY

The specialized strategies needed to extend a bibliotherapy program into clinical bibliotherapy are described more fully in chapter 2 and reinforced with a description of effective child therapy in chapter 5. These strategies include rapport-building and problem-exploration activities that precede a program of bibliotherapy, and follow-up and evaluation activities used subsequent to the program. In essence, these activities subsume a bibliotherapy program into a larger program of psychotherapy. When the decision is made to provide clinical rather than developmental bibliotherapy, one person should be designated as primarily responsible for ensuring that these additional steps are implemented.

9. EVALUATION

Upon completing a program of bibliotherapy, it is important to evaluate the degree to which the program's purposes have been achieved. Depending upon the purpose, this evaluation can occur through anecdotal reports by the children or their families, written rating forms or reports from others who know the child, direct observation of the child's new behavior, or a combination of these methods. Because the way in which a program is conducted can limit or make possible alternative methods of evaluation, it is important to determine in advance when and with what methods the program will be evaluated. In that way, important opportunities to collect program information will not be inadvertently overlooked. Assistance in planning an evaluation program, and in determining alternative evaluation resources to use, can be found in Rose and Edelson (1987).

The essential purpose of evaluation is to refine and improve the services that are offered to children and adolescents. Consequently, it is important that evaluation information be used to plan revised or supplementary activities for the next bibliotherapy program. Because each community has its own unique culture, becoming familiar with the types of activities that are successful in that community can be an invaluable legacy of an evaluation program.

SUMMARY

This nine-step planning process ensures that a program of bibliotherapy will be intentionally directed toward clear purposes, and so will have the best chance of success.

Such planning takes more time, initially, especially if it must occur within a team. Its ultimate efficiency is proven, though, when the resulting program proceeds more smoothly and more successfully than without such planning. To illustrate this planning process, as well as many of the other principles of this book, appendix B includes a program of bibliotherapy planned for fourth-graders to address issues of friendship and children in the class without friends.

REFERENCES

Conoley, J. C., and C. W. Conoley. 1992. *School Consultation: Practice and Training.* 2d ed. Boston: Allyn & Bacon.

Rose, S. D., and J. L. Edelson. 1987. *Working with Children and Adolescents in Groups.* San Francisco: Jossey-Bass Publishers.

APPENDIX A

Annotated Bibliography of Resources Containing Tips and Ideas for Bibliotherapy Activities

Bump, Jerome. 1990. "Innovative Bibliotherapy Approaches to Substance Abuse Education." *Arts in Psychotherapy* 17: 355–62.

This article provides a comprehensive description of a bibliotherapy program that has been successful with older adolescents. Discussions are included of initial selection of texts, strategies to focus on emotions and family dynamics, techniques for fostering effective small-group discussions, and selecting groups to be most effective. Bump is one of the few authors to report using computer-assisted class discussion strategies within his bibliotherapy program; he describes the advantages and pitfalls of these high-technology discussions. Although he focuses on issues of substance abuse, the strategies Bump describes could easily be applied to other high-risk behaviors of contemporary adolescents.

Gladding, Samuel T., and Claire Gladding. 1991. "The ABCs of Bibliotherapy for School Counselors." *School Counselor* (September): 7–13.

This article offers practical advice to professionals who plan to initiate a bibliotherapy program in schools. The Gladdings emphasize communicating clearly with the rest of the school community about what the program will be doing, when, and why. Then they provide specific tips on planning bibliotherapy sessions, including selecting appropriate rooms, developing and implementing strategies for fostering discussions, and creating a facilitative climate for the group. In particular, they show how to begin and end each group on a personal note.

Jeon, Kyung-Won. 1992. "Bibliotherapy for Gifted Children." *Gifted Child Today* (November/December): 16–19.

The last half of this article provides a summary of pragmatic tips for planning and conducting bibliotherapy programs. Included are suggested procedures for conducting after-reading discussions, questioning formats that facilitate reader reflection, and comprehension activities to reinforce readers' understandings of a book. Jeon also describes a five-step planning process to support bibliotherapy programs, and gives eight principles of bibliotherapy programs to guide leaders' decisions about how to proceed and with whom.

Pardeck, Jean A., and John T. Pardeck. 1984. "An Overview of the Bibliotherapeutic Treatment Approach: Implications for Clinical Social Work Practice." *Family Therapy* 11(3): 241–52.

Procedures for implementing clinical bibliotherapy programs are explained here, including sixteen different suggestions for creative writing, art, and discussion and role-playing activities that reinforce client understanding of a piece of literature.

Pardeck, Jean A., and John T. Pardeck, comps. 1986. "Books for Early Child-hood." *Bibliographies and Indexes in Psychology, Number 3.* New York: Greenwood Press.

In this book, the Pardecks give specific criteria for preschool bibliotherapy programs. Guidance is provided in selecting books, reading aloud, observing responses of preschoolers during the program, and conducting after-reading comprehension activities to reinforce preschoolers' understanding of a book's lessons.

Pardeck, John. 1994. "Using Literature to Help Adolescents Cope with Problems." *Adolescence* (Summer): 421–27.

Specific suggestions are provided for bibliotherapy programs targeting adolescents. In addition to providing creative strategies for reinforcing comprehension of literature, Pardeck lists specific books that he has used in different bibliotherapy programs.

Pardeck, John T., and Jean A. Pardeck. 1993. *Bibliotherapy: A Clinical Approach for Helping Children.* New York: Gordon and Breach Science Publishers.

This contemporary book includes discussions of the purposes, stages, and strategies appropriate for clinical bibliotherapy programs. Additionally, the authors have included a comprehensive list of books that are appropriate for children and youth, together with the typical ages of interest for each book.

Smith, Alice G. 1989. "Will the Real Bibliotherapist Please Stand Up?" *Journal of Youth Services in Libraries* (Spring): 241–49.

As a unique contribution, Smith provides a list of self-assessment questions for bibliotherapy leaders to use in evaluating their own skills. Questions are included regarding self-evaluation of one's group skills (e.g., "How do I motivate them into participation?"), selection of materials (e.g., "Are the books accurate in information about the topic?"), and selection of program location (e.g., "Is the room suitable for the use of media such as films and tapes?"). The result is a useful checklist of reminders for program leaders.

Sullivan, Joanna. 1987. "Read Aloud Sessions: Tackling Sensitive Issues Through Literature." *Reading Teacher* (May): 874–78.

Sullivan's tips describe important strategies for programs that intend to address controversial or sensitive topics. She describes ways of involving parents, selecting materials to use, conducting read-aloud sessions, and leading discussions. Finally, she provides specific, detailed examples of successful sessions she has used.

APPENDIX B

A Fourth-Grade Program in Children's Friendships

(Materials selected with the assistance of Jennifer Bowers.)

Problems with friends and recess are common in today's schools. For example, in one suburban fourth-grade classroom, students reported difficulties with arguing in 5 percent of their recesses, classmates refusing their requests to play in 4 percent of their recesses, problems being teased in 3 percent of recesses, and fighting in 1 percent of recesses (Doll and Murphy, 1996). Multiply these percentages by the 180 recess periods that most children have in a school year and it becomes apparent that most children will experience these or similar problems on at least a monthly basis. Similar rates of recess problems have been identified in other communities and classrooms. Rates this high tell us that problems with friends are unavoidable in childhood today. Consequently, the following bibliotherapy program has been developed to help this fourth-grade classroom decide how to handle the friendship problems that emerge on their playground.

While serving as an example of bibliotherapy for this book, the program is also being implemented in school as this book goes to press. Fourth-graders are gradually reading their way through several books from the selected materials and are engrossed in discussions about how their class will handle recess problems. Midprogram evaluation data have been collected and are promising—only a few of the students have been identified as needing more intensive therapeutic intervention.

TARGETED YOUTH

All fourth-grade students in a suburban elementary school of 720 students will participate in this Bibliotherapy Program. The program will be incorporated into the ongoing school day in their classroom. In the course of the program, students without friends may be identified and would then participate in a subsequent child therapy program about making and keeping friends.

PURPOSE OF THE PROGRAM

The purpose of this program is to reduce the number of problems that children in the class experience with friendships. When students in a class list their friends on a piece of paper, one or two children in every class will not be chosen by any of their classmates (Asher 1995). Students who have friendship difficulties that are frequent and enduring are at risk as adults to be unemployed or underemployed, lack independence, be overly aggressive, or experience serious mental health problems (Berndt 1984; Dodge 1989; Guralnick 1986). More immediately, having persistent and marked difficulties with friendships predisposes students to being removed from the class into special education programs (Hollinger 1987; Schonert-Reichl 1993) and causes children to be lonely and unhappy (Doll 1996). Recent research suggests that one effective way to help children with friendships may be to induce the entire peer group to be more flexible and accepting of classmates.

DECIDING UPON STAFFING

The principal leader of this bibliotherapy program will be the school psychologist in the elementary school. Classroom activities will be co-led with the fourth-grade teachers, and video and book materials have been selected in consultation with a children's librarian. The school psychologist was selected as principal leader because of her extensive clinical and research work on children's friendships. Moreover, if classroom-based activities are not successful in fostering friendships among those children who are currently without friends, the school psychologist will continue working with them, using individual child therapeutic programs that have successfully enhanced friendships in such children in previous research (Gettinger, Doll, and Salmon 1994).

CREATING THE PROFESSIONAL TEAM

The team relationship for this bibliotherapy program is essentially a consultative one. The school psychologist will request the assistance of the children's librarian throughout the program in reviewing and reevaluating the video and text materials used in the program.

SELECTED MATERIALS

The following materials have been selected to present ideas about children's friendships to the fourth-grade classroom. These were chosen to represent a range of reading levels, to include friendships of both boys and girls, and to represent a range of problems that might emerge among friends.

Novels

Adler, C. S. 1988. *Always and Forever Friends*. New York: Avon.
"If only Meg hadn't moved away. Then maybe eleven-year-old Wendy wouldn't be so upset about the other things going on in her life. Like her mother's marriage, and the new stepfamily that came with it. If only Wendy could find someone else like Meg to be her best friend—always and forever. There were the popular kids—who all stuck together—and there was Honor, a bright and interesting girl who didn't seem to want to be anybody's best friend. It was only when a new girl came into class and Wendy thought she'd found the perfect 'always and forever' friend that she really got to know Honor . . . and found out what friendship was all about" (from book cover). Contemporary realism. Grades 5–7.

Betancourt, Jeanne. 1993. *My Name is Brain Brian*. New York: Scholastic.
"When a tough new sixth-grade teacher focuses on Brian, Brian is sure he will be in trouble for the rest of his life. He is sure that now he will always be the class dummy. Then Brian finds out that the teacher doesn't think Brian is dumb. He thinks Brian has a learning difference: dyslexia. Before the school year is over, with the help of his teacher, Brian will have learned a whole new way of learning, as well as a whole new way of looking at the world, including his family, his friends, and himself" (from book jacket). Contemporary realism. Grades 4–6. Suggested passages to read aloud: pp. 54–55, friends influencing bad behavior; pp. 60–62, Brian and Dan question their relationship with their "best friends" and show fear about acting like their true selves; pp. 70–71, changing friendships; p. 5, Brian's journal entry.

Burch, Robert. 1982. *Ida Early Comes over the Mountain*. New York: Avon.
"Life was rough in the Blue Ridge Mountains of Georgia, but things certainly took a turn for the lively when Ida Early came over the mountain! For the four Sutton children, Ida appeared just in time. With their mother dead, their father at work, and unpredictable Ida hired on as housekeeper, bossy Aunt Ernestine might finally go back to Atlanta.
"Ida brought laughter back into the household. And the Suttons got used to her strange appearance and grew to love the tall tales she told at the toss of her hat. But their friendship was put to the test when the Sutton kids learned that there was more to Ida Early than just her funny ways" (from book cover). Child/adult friendship. Contemporary realism. Ages 9–12.

Byars, Betsy. 1981. *The Cybil War*. Illustrated by Gail Owens. New York: Viking Press.
"Simon learns some hard lessons about good and bad friendships when his good friend Tony's stories involve him in some very troublesome and complicated situations" (from CIP). At the same time, Simon has fallen in love with and is pursuing his schoolmate, Cybil. Contemporary realism. Easy reading. Ages 8–12.

Cassedy, Sylvia. 1987. *M.E. and Morton*. New York: Thomas Y. Crowell.
"Eleven-year-old Mary Ella, ashamed that her older brother Morton is a slow learner and longing for a friend of her own, is astonished when the flamboyant new girl on the block, [Polly], picks Morton for a friend" (from CIP). But Polly becomes Mary Ella's best friend as well. Contemporary realism. Ages 9–12. Suggested passages for reading aloud: pp. 20–29, M.E. is unsure how to initiate friendship; pp. 116–24, M.E. realizes that Polly likes Morton.

Conford, Ellen. 1992. *Anything for a Friend*. New York: Bantam Skylark (originally published by Little, Brown, 1979).
"Eleven-year-old Wallis Greene has had plenty of practice being the new girl in school. In fact, her family has moved so often that she should be used to it by now. But the truth is, trying to make friends and fit in never gets any easier. That's why, on her first day at Briar Lane Elementary School, Wallis decides to take the fast track to popularity by sticking close to Stuffy Sternwood, the class prankster. Wallis hopes that joining in Stuffy's crazy schemes will make the other kids like her. Then Stuffy's bright ideas start backfiring, and Wallis begins to wonder—just how far should she go to become popular?" (from book cover). Contemporary realism. Ages 9–11.

Elllis, Sarah. *Next-Door Neighbors.* New York: Margaret K. McElderry Books, 1990.
"Her family's move to a new town in Canada leaves the shy twelve-year-old Peggy feeling lonely and uncomfortable, until she befriends the unconventional George and the Chinese servant of the imperious neighbor Mrs. Manning" (from CIP). Contemporary realism. Grades 4–6. Suggested passages for reading aloud: pp. 20–24, in order to fit in and make friends at new school, Peggy tells a lie; pp. 44–47, Linda turns group against Peggy, and George, the class "weirdo," makes overtures; pp. 49–53, adult companionship/friendship with the servant, Sing.

Gaeddert, LouAnn. 1984. *Your Former Friend, Matthew.* Illustrated by Mary Beth Schwark. New York: Bantam Skylark.
"Gail and Matthew were best friends. They spent every day after school together. They shared their biggest secrets. They liked doing the same things. They even had the same thoughts at the same time. Then Matthew went away for the summer. And when he returned, he acted very strange. He stopped walking to school with Gail. And he started playing basketball with the boys all the time. He even forgot about the science fair project he promised to do with Gail! Gail found the change in Matthew very upsetting and puzzling. But she knew one thing—she had to do something to get her best friend back!" (from book cover). Contemporary realism. Easy reading. Ages 8–12.

Hall, Lynn. 1986. *Mrs. Portree's Pony.* New York: Charles Scribner's Sons.
"Addie, a foster child who feels unloved, seeks comfort in the company of a beautiful pony and begins an enriching relationship with its owner, a proud woman who has alienated and lost her own daughter" (from CIP). Child/adult friendship. Contemporary realism. Ages 9–12.

Hansen, Joyce. 1980. *The Gift-Giver.* New York: Houghton Mifflin.
"Amir, a gentle loner, is the new boy on the block. Doris is amazed that he doesn't seem to care about doing what everyone else does. As Doris and Amir become friends, he helps her to grow in self-confidence and in her understanding of others. When her father loses his job, it is Amir's influence that enables Doris to play an active role in keeping her family together—even though it means growing apart from her friends" (from book jacket). Multicultural title. Contemporary realism. Grades 4–7. Suggested passages to read aloud: pp. 54–55, trying to fit in yet also be comfortable with being different from the group; pp. 71–81, learning to accept outsiders; pp. 109–14, group realizes how much Amir means to them once he has gone.

Hansen, Joyce. 1986. *Yellow Bird and Me.* New York: Clarion Books.
"It's only been a few weeks since Amir's foster family took him away from his friends in the Bronx and placed him in a group home in Syracuse, New York. Doris doesn't think she'll ever get used to his being gone, though. Her friends on 163rd Street are no substitute for Amir—especially not that silly 'Yellow Bird' (from book jacket). But Yellow Bird persists, and he and Doris become good friends. Multicultural title. Contemporary realism. Grades 4–6. Suggested passages to read aloud: pp. 64–69, Doris helps Bird as a way to reconnect with Amir; pp. 101–5, Doris genuinely begins to care about Bird. Note: It may be best to share *The Gift-Giver* with the audience first, so that they understand Doris's friendship with Amir.

Konigsburg, E. L. 1967. *Jennifer, Hecate, Macbeth, William McKinley, and Me, Elizabeth*. New York: Atheneum.

"Elizabeth is the loneliest child in the whole U.S. of A. until she discovers Jennifer. Of course, Jennifer isn't a friend, really. Witches don't make friends, and Jennifer is a witch. Elizabeth becomes her apprentice, however, and in the process of learning how to become a witch herself, she also learns how to eat raw eggs, how to cast short spells, and how to get along with Jennifer, among other things" (from book jacket). Contemporary realism. Grades 4–6.

Lisle, Janet Taylor. 1989. *Afternoon of the Elves*. New York: Orchard Books.

"Everyone warned Hillary about Sara-Kate Connolly, the sullen, too-thin girl who lived in a dilapidated house down the hill. 'She's too old for you,' her friends said. 'She's definitely not a person you can trust. Stay away from her.' But how could Hillary, nine, stay away from the delicate stick houses, 'small enough for mice,' that appeared one day in Sara-Kate's junky backyard?" (from book jacket). Newbery Honor book. Contemporary realism. Grades 4–6. Suggested passages to read aloud: pp. 2–33, beginning of friendship between Hillary and Sara-Kate; pp. 3–64, Hillary defends her friend; pp. 109–13, Hillary expresses doubts about her friendship with Sara-Kate.

Lowry, Lois. 1989. *Number the Stars*. Boston: Houghton Mifflin.

"As the German troops begin their campaign to 'relocate' all the Jews of Denmark, the Johansens take in Annemarie's best friend, Ellen Rosen, and pretend she is part of the family. Ellen and Annemarie must think quickly when three Nazi officers arrive late one night and question why Ellen is not blond, like her sisters" (from book jacket). Newbery Medal winner. Historical fiction. Grades 4+.

Madison, Winifred. *Marinka, Katinka, and Me (Susie)*. Pictures by Miller Pope. Scarsdale, NY: Bradbury Press, 1975.

"Marinka, Katinka, and Susie are friends. . . . Three happens to be the lucky number for jumping rope (or dancing a special dance in the class play), so when, one day, Marinka gets mad at Katinka, all sorts of plans and fun are wrecked. Susie is struck by something about friendship: friends can end up strangers if they stop talking with each other . . ." (from book jacket). Contemporary realism. Ages 7–10. Suggested passages for reading aloud: pp. 6–7, description of what it's like to have friends; pp. 49–52, a fight between friends results in one person being excluded from the trio.

Moore, Emily. *Whose Side Are You On?* New York: Farrar, Straus & Giroux, 1988.

"Barbra can't believe her bad luck. First her sixth-grade teacher fails her in math. Then she is assigned T.J. Brodie—the pest—as a tutor. But when they study together, Barbra sees a side of T.J. that is patient and serious, and much to her surprise, she begins to like him" (from book jacket). Multicultural title. Contemporary realism. Grades 4–6. Suggested passages for reading aloud: pp. 84–86, threesome dynamics; pp. 122–24, Barbra sticks up for the outsider and consequently she is ostracized from the group.

Myers, Walter Dean. 1988. *Scorpions*. New York: Harper & Row.
"The only one who understands is Tito, Jamal's best friend. It is Tito who shares long walks from Harlem to the boat basin; who argues about which of them will have the bigger boat when they're rich; who admires Jamal's drawings. It is Tito who joins the Scorpions when Jamal takes over, in spite of his fear, so he can look out for his friend. Then Angel and Indian challenge Jamal's position as leader of the Scorpions, calling him to a showdown in the park. But when Angel pulls out a knife, Tito acts to save his friend and nearly destroys his own life. The trouble is, even though Jamal can see that everything about the gun is bad, a part of him that is small and afraid still wants it" (from book jacket). Newbery Honor book. Multicultural title. Contemporary realism. Grades 5–10.

Namioka, Lensey. 1992. *Yang the Youngest and His Terrible Ear*. Illustrated by Kees de Kiefte. Boston: Little, Brown.
"Recently arrived in Seattle from China, musically untalented Yingtao is faced with giving a violin performance to attract new students for his father when he would rather be working on friendships and playing baseball" (from CIP). Multicultural title. Contemporary realism. Grades 4–7.

Paterson, Katherine. 1977. *Bridge to Terabithia*. Illustrated by Donna Diamond. New York: Thomas Crowell.
"Somewhat to Jess's surprise, he and Leslie became friends, and the worlds of imagination and learning that she opened up to him changed him forever. It was Leslie's idea to create Terabithia, their secret kingdom in the woods where they reigned supreme. There no enemy—not their teacher Monster Mouth Myers, their schoolmates Gary Fulcher and Janice Avery, Jess's four sisters, or even Jess's own fears and Leslie's imaginary foes—could defeat them. The legacy that Leslie finally brought to Jess enabled him to cope with the unexpected tragedy that touched them all" (from book jacket). Newbery Award winner. Contemporary realism. Grades 4+.

Paterson, Katherine. 1994. *Flip-Flop Girl*. New York: Lodestar Books.
"Living with Grandma in Brownsville, Virginia, means going to the Gertrude B. Spitzer Elementary School, where all the girls in their pretty, new clothes ask why her brother Mason is so crazy. Only Mr. Clayton, Vinnie's handsome young teacher, makes school bearable. But at recess time, Vinnie sees a tall, lanky girl playing hopscotch alone, and her curiosity gets the best of her. Why does Lupe wear bright orange flip-flops? And why is she always getting into trouble? In the midst of her anger and confusion, Vinnie finds a rare friendship—and very nearly destroys it" (from book jacket). Contemporary realism. Grades 4–6.

Peck, Robert Newton. 1974. *Soup*. Illustrated by Charles C. Gehm. New York: Alfred A. Knopf.
Here are the stories of a friendship between two boys in Vermont—"stories from a boyhood filled with barrels to roll in, apples to whip, windows to break, ropes to bind prisoners, acorn pipes, and ten-cent Saturday movies. It was a time when the days seemed a little bit longer; life a little simpler. But then as always nothing was quite as important as a best friend" (from book jacket). Historical fiction. Grades 5+.

Rylant, Cynthia. 1986. *A Fine White Dust*. New York: Bradbury Press.

"The visit of the traveling Preacher Man to his small North Carolina town gives new impetus to thirteen-year-old Peter's struggle to reconcile his own deeply felt religious belief with the beliefs and nonbeliefs of his family and friends" (from CIP). Contemporary realism. Grades 5+.

Slepian, Jan. 1980. *The Alfred Summer*. New York: Macmillan.

"Saving Alfred's life was the real beginning for Lester. Of course he didn't actually save Alfred. He just stood there on the beach, desperately trying to sound the alarm, unable to get the words out, unable even to point to the danger. But he *helped*, and he found a friend at last. So what if Alfred is retarded? He's special anyway, the only person Lester has ever met who is the same on the inside as he is on the outside. He doesn't seem to notice or care that Lester has cerebral palsy. Besides, without Alfred, Lester would never have known about the getaway boat" (from book jacket). Historical fiction. Grades 5+.

Slepian, Jan. 1981. *Lester's Turn*. New York: Macmillan.

In this "stunning sequel to Jan Slepian's critically acclaimed first novel, *The Alfred Summer,* everything has changed since that fateful summer and none of it good as far as 16-year-old Lester is concerned. Worst of all is watching his retarded friend Alfie waste away in the hospital. Lester, himself a cerebral palsy victim, is desperate to save Alfie, and from this desperation is born the daring—but disastrous—kidnapping attempt" (from book jacket). Historical fiction. Ages 11–14.

Smith, Doris Buchanan. 1991. *The Pennywhistle Tree*. New York: G. P. Putnam's Sons.

"A rift develops in the closeness shared by eleven-year-old Jonathon and his best friends when a new boy moves onto the street and insists on pushing himself into Jonathon's life" (from CIP). Contemporary realism. Grades 4–6.

Snyder, Zilpha Keatley. 1967. *The Egypt Game*. Drawings by Alton Raible. New York: Atheneum.

"Even to Melanie, who knew that you could never predict what a new kid would be like, April Hall was something of a surprise. One look at her stringy upswept hair, false eyelashes, and ragged fox fur collar, convinced Melanie that April was not going to be easy to integrate into the sixth grade at Jackson School. But April had other surprises to offer, like the fact that she enjoyed reading and loved playing imagination games just as much as Melanie. Within a month April and Melanie had developed a common interest in ancient Egypt and had begun to develop a land of Egypt in an abandoned storage yard" (from book jacket). Contemporary realism. Grades 5–7.

Stolz, Mary. 1965. *The Noonday Friends*. Illustrated by Lois S. Glanzman. New York: Harper Trophy.

"Franny wants her sandwich packed in a lunch box or even a paper bag. Anything but a free lunch pass. She also wants to be able to spend time with her best friend, Simone, outside the cafeteria, after school. But Franny's charming artist father can't seem to hold a job, and her mother works full time; so the eleven-year-old New Yorker has a lot of responsibilities and worries at home. Because Simone often has to help out in her own large immigrant family, she understands, most of the time. But lately Franny thinks wealthy Lila has more to offer Simone . . ." (from book cover). Newbery Honor book. Contemporary realism. Grades 4–6.

Taha, Karen T. *A Gift for Tia Rosa*. Illustrated by Dee deRosa. Minneapolis, MN: Dillon Press, 1986.

"Little Carmela is close to her elderly neighbor and saddened by her illness and death, but she finds a way to express her love when Tia Rosa's grandchild is born" (from CIP). Multicultural title. Child/adult friendship. Contemporary realism. Grades 3–4.

Willis, Meredith Sue. 1994. *The Secret Super Powers of Marco*. New York: Harper Trophy.

"Marco has Special Powers. He uses them to save his dog, to find his sister, and to help his new friend Tyrone get a job. Marco's mama thinks Tyrone is destined for a life of crime. Only Marco sees something else in Tyrone. He sees the good beneath the bully, and a true friend" (from book cover). Contemporary realism. Easy reading. Ages 8–12.

Picture Books

Fleischman, Sid. 1987. *The Scarebird*. Pictures by Peter Sis. New York: Greenwillow Books.

"A lonely old farmer realizes the value of human friendship when a young man comes to help him and his scarecrow with their farm" (from CIP).

Keats, Ezra Jack. 1971. *Apt. 3*. New York: Macmillan.

"On a day when rain softens the sounds of the city, Sam hears someone in his building playing the harmonica. Curious, he and his little brother try to find out where the music is coming from. What the boys discover is beautiful and surprising—not just music or a new friend, but something unexpected within themselves" (from book jacket).

Lobel, Arnold. 1970. *Frog and Toad Are Friends*. New York: Harper & Row.

This title, as well as other Frog and Toad books, presents the daily activities of two friends and shows how they nurture and maintain their friendship.

Marshall, James. 1972. *George and Martha*. Boston: Houghton Mifflin.

"Friendship proves a delicate thing, even when it exists between two not so delicate creatures as George and Martha. Loving and lovable a hippopotamus might well be, but delicate he is not. Even so, George and Martha seem to know full well the joys and delights of having a friend to cheer you and care, someone who will tell you the truth and go to great lengths to spare your feelings" (from book jacket).

Naylor, Phyllis Reynolds. *King of the Playground*. Illustrated by Nola Langner Malone. New York: Atheneum, 1991.

"Kevin loves to go to the playground, but not when Sammy is there. . . . And then one day Kevin gets his courage up and goes to the playground even though Sammy says he can't come in. . . . Will Kevin stay, or will he go home? How will he deal with Sammy?" (from book jacket).

Polacco, Patricia. 1992. *Chicken Sunday*. New York: Philomel Books.

" 'Stewart and Winston were my neighbors. They were my brothers by a solemn ceremony we had performed in their backyard one summer. . . . Their gramma, Eula Mae Walker, was my gramma now.' More than anything in the world, the children want to buy that special Easter bonnet in Mr. Kodinski's shop window for their Miss Eula. . . . But the hat costs money and the children do not have enough. Then one day, when they are mistakenly accused of throwing eggs at the shopowner's window, they discover just the right way to prove their innocence— and earn money for the hat at the same time" (from book jacket).

Rylant, Cynthia. 1983. *Miss Maggie*. Illustrated by Thomas DiGrazia. New York: E. P. Dutton.

Nat Crawford was always trying to peer in one of Miss Maggie's windows to see the black snake that folks said hung from the rafters inside. "[H]e had to peek through a window, or the doorway, because he didn't ever want to go inside old Miss Maggie's cabin. And then one winter something happened to Miss Maggie. What Nat does to help her makes a rich and memorable story about a very special person" (from book jacket).

Steptoe, John. 1969. *Stevie*. New York: Harper & Row.

"One day Robert's mother told him, 'You know you're gonna have a little friend come stay with you.' So little Stevie came. And right away he was nothing but a pest. He'd break Robert's toys and get him in trouble. All the time he got in the way with his old spoiled self. But then one day Stevie's mother and father came to take him away for good. Soon Robert began thinking maybe Stevie wasn't so bad after all" (from book jacket).

Viorst, Judith. 1974. *Rosie and Michael*. Illustrated by Lorna Tomei. New York: Atheneum.

"Friendship overcomes all problems. That's what Rosie and Michael think. It's big enough for jokes, for laughter, for sharing possessions, for aiding each other in dire emergencies, and even for being mad once in a while" (from book jacket).

Waber, Bernard. 1972. *Ira Sleeps Over*. Boston: Houghton Mifflin.

" 'I was invited to sleep at Reggie's house. Was I happy! I had never slept at a friend's house before.' And with an agenda for the evening that includes a special showing of the junk collection, a wrestling match, a pillow fight, magic tricks, checkers, dominoes, a magnifying glass, and ghost stories, who wouldn't be excited? In the end and in an entirely unexpected way, however, the night proves to be a happier one than even Ira could have imagined" (from book jacket).

Winners of the Parade-Kodak National Photo Contest. *Best Friends: A Pictorial Celebration*. Introduction by Waller Anderson. New York: Continuum Publishing, 1991.

"When Parade and Kodak announced their contest for photographs of Best Friends, they received more than 200,000 entries—the most ever. And the best friends represented in these photographs transcend age, race, sex and even species" (from book jacket).

Poetry

Livingston, Myra Cohn, ed. 1987. *I Like You, If You Like Me: Poems of Friendship*. New York: Margaret K. McElderry Books.

"The sadness of solitude; the tentative exploration of new and blossoming friendships; the joy of a faithful pet to whom all troubles can be confided and of make-believe friends and best friends; the painful moments, too, of fighting and reconciling, of parting and being reunited are among the many acts of friendship shared here through poetry" (from book jacket). This anthology includes the work of ninety traditional and contemporary poets.

Schenk de Regniers, Beatrice. 1986. *A Week in the Life of Best Friends and Other Poems of Friendship*. Illustrated by Nancy Doyle. New York: Atheneum.

"[F]riends are sometimes nearby and sometimes not, sometimes loyal and sometimes not, sometimes helpful and sometimes not, sometimes other children and sometimes a pet or even a bee. And once in a while there is someone who wonders if being alone is not important, too" (from book jacket).

Audiovisual Materials

Bridge to Terabithia. 1985. 58 minutes. Color. Produced by Wonderworks, distributed by Public Media Video. Ages 9–13.

Live-action drama filmed in Canada dramatizes Katherine Patterson's book of the same title (see prior entry). The only variation from the original title finds Jesse blaming himself for his friend's death. Moss and Wilson 1992, pp. 45–46.

Frog and Toad Are Friends. 1985. 17.5 minutes. Color. Animated. Produced by John Matthews for Churchill Media. Ages 4–8.

Three-dimensional animation portrays the friendship of Frog and Toad as shown in Lobel's book of the same title. See comments in the entry under "Picture Books." Other titles in the series have also been animated. Moss and Wilson 1992, p. 100.

Soup and Me. 1977. 24 minutes. Color. Produced by ABC Weekend Specialists, distributed by Coronet/MTI Film and Video. Ages 8–11.

From Robert Newton Peck's book of the same title, this film follows the escapades of two young boys. Peck based the book on his own childhood and best friend in rural Vermont. *Soup for President* is also available. Moss and Wilson 1992, p. 310.

COMPREHENSION ACTIVITIES

Beginning in September, the school psychologist will read a book selected from the list to the class during the twenty minutes of oral reading scheduled to occur every day after recess. The book will be selected with the teachers' suggestions. As the students in the class become accustomed to having the school psychologist join them in class, the daily reading selection will be followed by a brief discussion of one or two issues of friendship that emerged during that day's reading.

In early October, the school psychologist and teachers will conduct a meeting with the class to brainstorm a list of the things students want to know about friendships and making and keeping friends. Additional materials will be selected from the list when they match the questions that the class raises about friendships. These books and films will be infused into classroom activities in one or more of the following ways:

1. Students will read them as part of the regularly scheduled reading instruction.

2. The class members will view the film or a brief picture book as a prompt for writing activities, including writing about the most difficult problem they had with a friend, their best friend, what makes a person a good friend, or what to do to solve problems with friends.

3. Students will read poetry about friendships and then write their own poetry for greeting cards meant for friends.

In early November, the school psychologist and classroom teachers will host a second class meeting with the students. The purpose of this meeting will be to identify any problems that students are struggling with concerning recess. These problems will be listed on a brief questionnaire and, beginning with the first meeting, immediately after coming back into the classroom, students will circle the problems they had difficulty with during that day's recess. These recess reports will be tabulated and graphed as part of the class's math lesson.

Students will continue to read or listen to the bibliotherapy selections as before, but now they will be looking for other examples of the class's most prevalent problems. When examples are found, the strategies that fictional characters use to solve them will be added to a giant list of solutions on the classroom's bulletin board. Each week, the class will review these solutions, and choose from them to write an action plan to solve some of the class friendship problems.

EXTENSIONS REQUIRED BY CLINICAL BIBLIOTHERAPY

Should some students continue to need additional assistance with friendships, the school psychologist will employ a program of systematic social problem solving (Elias and Tobias 1996) and personal goal setting (Gettinger, Doll, and Salmon 1994). These strategies have proven effective in assisting children with friendships in prior research.

EVALUATION

The class recess reports will serve as a useful indicator of the success of this bibliotherapy program. In addition, reports from those students who had no friends will show whether these students' problems with friends have improved, worsened, or stayed the same.

REFERENCES

Asher, S. R. 1995. "Children and Adolescents with Peer Relationship Problems." A workshop presented at the Annual Summer Institute in School Psychology: Internalizing Disorders in Children and Adolescents. Denver, Colorado, June.

Berndt, T. J. 1984. "Sociometric, Socio-cognitive and Behavioral Measures for the Study of Friendship and Popularity." In *Friendship in Normal and Handicapped Children,* ed. T. Field, J. L. Roopnarine, and M. Segal. Norwood, NJ: Ablex, pp. 31–45.

Dodge, K. A. 1989. "Problems in Social Relationships." In *Treatment of Childhood Disorders,* ed. E. J. Mash and R. A. Barkley. New York: Guilford Press, pp. 222–46.

Doll, B. 1996. "Children Without Friends: Implications for Practice and Policy." *School Psychology Review* 25: 165–83.

Doll, B., and P. Murphy. 1996. "Recess Reports: Self-identification of Students with Friendship Difficulties." A paper presented at the 104th Annual Convention of the American Psychological Association. Toronto, Ontario.

Elias, M. J., and S. E. Tobias. 1996. *Social Problem Solving: Interventions in the Schools.* New York: Guilford Press.

Gettinger, M., B. Doll, and D. Salmon. 1994. "Effects of Social Problem-solving, Goal-setting, and Parent Training on Children's Peer Relations." *Journal of Applied Developmental Psychology* 15: 141–63.

Guralnick, M. 1986. "The Peer Relations of Young Handicapped and Nonhandicapped Children." In *Children's Social Behavior: Development, Assessment and Modification,* ed. P. Straim, M. Guralnick, and H. M. Walker. New York: Academic Press, pp. 93–140.

Hollinger, J. D. 1987. "Social Skills for Behaviorally Disordered Children as Preparation for Mainstreaming: Theory, Practice and New Directions." *Remedial and Special Education* 8: 17–27.

Moss, Joyce, and George Wilson, eds. 1992. *From Page to Screen: Children's and Young Adults' Books on Film and Video.* Detroit: Gale Research.

Schonert-Reichl, K. A. 1993. "Empathy and Social Relationships in Adolescents with Behavioral Disorders." *Behavior Disorders* 18: 189–204.

INDEX